Sleep, Memory, and Learning

Guest Editor

ROBERT STICKGOLD, PhD

SLEEP MEDICINE CLINICS

www.sleep.theclinics.com

March 2011 • Volume 6 • Number 1

SAUNDERS an imprint of ELSEVIER, Inc.

W.B. SAUNDERS COMPANY
A Division of Elsevier Inc.

1600 John F. Kennedy Boulevard ● Suite 1800 ● Philadelphia, PA 19103-2899

http://www.sleep.theclinics.com

SLEEP MEDICINE CLINICS Volume 6, Number 1
March 2011, ISSN 1556-407X, ISBN-13: 978-1-4557-0504-7

Editor: Sarah E. Barth
Developmental Editor: Jessica Demetriou

Sleep Medicine Clinics (ISSN 1556-407X) is published quarterly by Elsevier Inc., 360 Park Avenue South, New York, NY 10010-1710. Months of issue are March, June, September and December. Business and Editorial Offices: 1600 John F. Kennedy Blvd., Ste. 1800, Philadelphia, PA 19103-2899. Customer Service Office: 3251 Riverport Lane, Maryland Heights, MO 63043. Periodicals postage paid at New York, NY and additional mailing offices. Subscription prices are $161.00 per year (US individuals), $80.00 (US residents), $346.00 (US institutions), $198.00 (foreign individuals), $111.00 (foreign residents), and $381.00 (foreign institutions). Foreign air speed delivery is included in all *Clinics* subscription prices. All prices are subject to change without notice. **POSTMASTER:** Send change of address to *Sleep Medicine Clinics*, Elsevier Health Sciences Division, Subscription Customer Service, 3251 Riverport Lane, Maryland Heights, MO 63043. Customer Service: **Tel: 1-800-654-2452 (U.S. and Canada); 314-447-8871 (outside U.S. and Canada). Fax: 314-447-8029. E-mail: journalscustomerservice-usa@elsevier.com (for print support); journalsonlinesupport-usa@elsevier.com (for online support).**

Reprints. For copies of 100 or more of articles in this publication, please contact the Commercial Reprints Department, Elsevier Inc., 360 Park Avenue South, New York, NY 10010-1710. Tel.: 212-633-3812; Fax: 212-462-1935; E-mail: reprints@elsevier.com.

Printed and bound in the United Kingdom
Transferred to Digital Print 2011

GOAL STATEMENT

The goal of *Sleep Clinics of North America* is to keep practicing physicians up to date with current clinical practice by providing timely articles reviewing the state of the art in patient care.

ACCREDITATION

The *Sleep Clinics of North America* is planned and implemented in accordance with the Essential Areas and Policies of the Accreditation Council for Continuing Medical Education (ACCME) through the joint sponsorship of the University of Virginia School of Medicine and Elsevier. The University of Virginia School of Medicine is accredited by the ACCME to provide continuing medical education for physicians.

The University of Virginia School of Medicine designates this educational activity for a maximum of 15 *AMA PRA Category 1 Credits*™ for each issue, 60 credits per year. Physicians should only claim credit commensurate with the extent of their participation in the activity.

The American Medical Association has determined that physicians not licensed in the US who participate in this CME activity are eligible for a maximum of 15 *AMA PRA Category 1 Credits*™ for each issue, 60 credits per year.

Credit can be earned by reading the text material, taking the CME examination online at http://www.theclinics.com/home/cme, and completing the evaluation. After taking the test, you will be required to review any and all incorrect answers. Following completion of the test and evaluation, your credit will be awarded and you may print your certificate.

FACULTY DISCLOSURE/CONFLICT OF INTEREST

The University of Virginia School of Medicine, as an ACCME accredited provider, endorses and strives to comply with the Accreditation Council for Continuing Medical Education (ACCME) Standards of Commercial Support, Commonwealth of Virginia statutes, University of Virginia policies and procedures, and associated federal and private regulations and guidelines on the need for disclosure and monitoring of proprietary and financial interests that may affect the scientific integrity and balance of content delivered in continuing medical education activities under our auspices.

The University of Virginia School of Medicine requires that all CME activities accredited through this institution be developed independently and be scientifically rigorous, balanced and objective in the presentation/discussion of its content, theories and practices.

All authors/editors participating in an accredited CME activity are expected to disclose to the readers relevant financial relationships with commercial entities occurring within the past 12 months (such as grants or research support, employee, consultant, stock holder, member of speakers bureau, etc.). The University of Virginia School of Medicine will employ appropriate mechanisms to resolve potential conflicts of interest to maintain the standards of fair and balanced education to the reader. Questions about specific strategies can be directed to the Office of Continuing Medical Education, University of Virginia School of Medicine, Charlottesville, Virginia.

The faculty and staff of the University of Virginia Office of Continuing Medical Education have no financial affiliations to disclose.

The authors/editors listed below have identified no professional or financial affiliations for themselves or their spouse/partner:

Ted Abel, PhD; Sarah Barth (Acquisitions Editor); Jan Born, PhD; Jennifer H. Breslin, MA; Cynthia Brown, MD (Test Author); Jason K.M. Chau, MD, MPH, FRCS(C); Rebecca L. Gomez, MA, PhD; Pepe J. Hernandez, PhD; Lisa Marshall, PhD; Katherine C. Newman-Smith, BA; Louise M. O'Brien, PhD; Nelson B. Powell, MD, DDS; Carlyle Smith, PhD; Els van der Helm, MSc; Matthew P. Walker, PhD; and Erin J. Wamsley, PhD.

The authors/editors listed below identified the following professional or financial affiliations for themselves or their spouse/partner:

Richard R. Bootzin, MS, PhD is an industry funded research/investigator for Takeda Phamaceuticals, and is a consultant for Consolidated Research.
Teofilo Lee-Chiong Jr, MD (Consulting Editor) is an industry funded research/investigator for Respironics and Embla.
Jessica D. Payne, PhD is a consultant and is on the Advisory Board/Committee for Humana, Inc.
Robert Stickgold, PhD (Guest Editor) is a consultant for Eli Lilly.
Todd J. Swick, MD is an industry funded researcher and is on the Speakers' Bureau for Sunovian and Somaxon, is an industry funded researcher for Teva, and is an industry funded researcher and consultant, and is on the Speakers' Bureau and Advisory Board for Jazz Pharmaceuticals.

Disclosure of Discussion of Non-FDA Approved Uses for Pharmaceutical Products and/or Medical Devices.

The University of Virginia School of Medicine, as an ACCME provider, requires that all faculty presenters identify and disclose any off-label uses for pharmaceutical and medical device products. The University of Virginia School of Medicine recommends that each physician fully review all the available data on new products or procedures prior to clinical use.

TO ENROLL

To enroll in the Sleep Clinics of North America Continuing Medical Education program, call customer service at 1-800-654-2452 or visit us online at www.theclinics.com/home/cme. The CME program is available to subscribers for an additional fee of $114.00.

Sleep Medicine Clinics

FORTHCOMING ISSUES

June 2011

Genetics and Sleep
Allan Pack, MD, *Guest Editor*

September 2011

Portable Sleep Monitoring
Michael R. Littner, MD,
Guest Editor

December 2011

Parasomnias
Mark R. Pressman, PhD, *Guest Editor*

RECENT ISSUES

December 2010

Medications and Sleep
Timothy Roehrs, PhD, *Guest Editor*

September 2010

Positive Airway Pressure Therapy
Richard B. Berry, MD,
Guest Editor

June 2010

Dreaming and Nightmares
J.F. Pagel, MS, MD, *Guest Editor*

THE CLINICS ARE NOW AVAILABLE ONLINE!

Access your subscription at:
www.theclinics.com

Contributors

CONSULTING EDITOR

TEOFILO LEE-CHIONG Jr, MD
Professor of Medicine and Chief, Division
of Sleep Medicine, National Jewish Health;
Associate Professor of Medicine, University
of Colorado Denver School of Medicine,
Denver, Colorado

GUEST EDITOR

ROBERT STICKGOLD, PhD
Associate Professor of Psychiatry, Center for
Sleep and Cognition, Beth Israel Deaconess
Medical Center; and Harvard Medical School,
Boston, Massachusetts

AUTHORS

TED ABEL, PhD
Brush Family Professor of Biology; Director,
Biological Basis of Behavior Program,
Department of Biology, University of
Pennsylvania, Lynch Laboratories,
Philadelphia, Pennsylvania

RICHARD R. BOOTZIN, MS, PhD
Psychology Department, The University
of Arizona, Tucson, Arizona

JAN BORN, PhD
Department of Neuroendocrinology, University
of Lübeck, Lübeck; Institute of Pyschology and
Behavioral Neurobiology, University of
Tübingen, Tübingen, Germany

JENNIFER H. BRESLIN, MA
Psychology Department, The University
of Arizona, Tucson, Arizona

JASON K.M. CHAU, MD, MPH, FRCS(C)
Assistant Professor, Department of
Otolaryngology Head and Neck Surgery,
University of Manitoba, Winnipeg, Manitoba,
Canada

REBECCA L. GOMEZ, MA, PhD
Psychology Department, The University
of Arizona, Tucson, Arizona

PEPE J. HERNANDEZ, PhD
Postdoctoral Fellow, Department of Biology,
University of Pennsylvania, Lynch
Laboratories, Philadelphia, Pennsylvania

LISA MARSHALL, PhD
Department of Neuroendocrinology, University
of Lübeck, Lübeck, Germany

KATHARINE C. NEWMAN-SMITH, BA
Psychology Department, The University
of Arizona, Tucson, Arizona

LOUISE M. O'BRIEN, PhD
Assistant Professor, Sleep Disorders Center,
Department of Neurology, University
of Michigan, Ann Arbor; Department of Oral
and Maxillofacial Surgery, University
of Michigan, Ann Arbor, Michigan

JESSICA D. PAYNE, PhD
Assistant Professor of Psychology,
Department of Psychology, University of Notre
Dame, Notre Dame, Indiana

NELSON B. POWELL, MD, DDS, FACS
Adjunct Clinical Professor, Department
of Otolaryngology Head and Neck Surgery;
Department of Psychiatry and Behavioral
Science, Stanford University Sleep and
Research Center, Stanford University
School of Medicine, Palo Alto, Stanford,
California

CARLYLE SMITH, PhD
Professor Emeritus of Psychology, Department
of Psychology, Trent University, Peterborough,
Ontario, Canada

ROBERT STICKGOLD, PhD
Associate Professor of Psychiatry, Center for
Sleep and Cognition, Beth Israel Deaconess
Medical Center; and Harvard Medical School,
Boston, Massachusetts

TODD J. SWICK, MD
Assistant Clinical Professor of Neurology,
School of Medicine, University of
Texas-Houston; and Medical Director,
The Houston Sleep Center, Houston, Texas

ELS VAN DER HELM, MSc
Sleep and Neuroimaging Laboratory,
Department of Psychology and Helen Wills
Neuroscience Institute, University of California,
Berkeley, California

MATTHEW P. WALKER, PhD
Sleep and Neuroimaging Laboratory,
Department of Psychology and Helen Wills
Neuroscience Institute, University of California,
Berkeley, California

ERIN J. WAMSLEY, PhD
Instructor in Psychiatry, Department of
Psychiatry, Beth Israel Deaconess Medical
Center; and Harvard Medical School, Boston,
Massachusetts

Contents

Foreword   xi

Teofilo Lee-Chiong Jr

Preface: Sleep, Learning, and Memory   xiii

Robert Stickgold

The Neurology of Sleep   1

Todd J. Swick

> Neurology, by virtue of its study of the brain, is the primary medical science for the elucidation of the anatomy, physiology, pathology and ultimately, the function of sleep. There has been nothing short of a revolution in the science of sleep over the past 50 years. From the discovery of REM sleep to the identification of Hypocretin/Orexin the basic science and clinical field of sleep medicine has blossomed. This article will explore the anatomy, physiology, biochemistry and, to a limited extent, pathophysiology of the sleep/wake centers of the brain. The field of chronobiology will also be touched upon.

Learning, Memory, and Sleep in Humans   15

Jessica D. Payne

> In spite of advances in understanding the processes that generate and maintain sleep, the functional significance of sleep remains a mystery. Numerous theories regarding sleep's function have been proposed, including homeostatic restoration, thermoregulation, tissue repair, and immune control, but the theory that has received enormous attention in the last decade concerns sleep's role in processing and storing memories. This article reviews evidence that sleep is critical for long-lasting memories. Although this article mostly focuses on memory consolidation, it also briefly reviews new evidence that sleep is essential for effective memory encoding.

Sleep and Emotional Memory Processing   31

Els van der Helm and Matthew P. Walker

> Cognitive neuroscience continues to build meaningful connections between affective behavior and human brain function. Within the biologic sciences, a similar renaissance has taken place, focusing on the role of sleep in various neurocognitive processes, and most recently, the interaction between sleep and emotional regulation. This review surveys an array of diverse findings across basic and clinical research domains, resulting in a convergent view of sleep-dependent emotional brain processing. Based on the unique neurobiology of sleep, the authors outline a model describing the overnight modulation of affective neural systems and the (re)processing of recent emotional experiences.

Learning, Memory, and Sleep in Children   45

Rebecca L. Gomez, Katharine C. Newman-Smith, Jennifer H. Breslin, and Richard R. Bootzin

> This article reviews research on the effects of sleep quality on cognitive outcomes in infancy, childhood, and adolescence; the effects of sleep restriction on cognitive

measures in children; and experimental studies investigating differences in memory consolidation in sleep and wake states after learning in infant, child, and adolescent populations. The studies point to an essential role for sleep in cognitive development, with many similarities between the effects of sleep on learning in children and adults and some surprising differences. Achieving adequate sleep may be particularly important to higher level cognitive functioning in early childhood.

Sleep States and Memory Processing in Rodents: A Review   59

Carlyle Smith

That there is a relationship between sleep states and memory consolidation is now well established. Studies are now focused on exactly how sleep is related to other known memory mechanisms. Technological advances have allowed investigators to observe brain activity at the cellular and intracellular levels in various brain structures during sleep at different posttraining times. The experiments described provide detailed data at the electrophysiologic, neurophysiologic, and neurochemical levels. A comprehensive understanding of the exact nature of sleep-memory mechanisms requires the incorporation of all of these findings.

A Molecular Basis for Interactions Between Sleep and Memory   71

Pepe J. Hernandez and Ted Abel

The electrophysiological properties of the sleeping brain profoundly influence memory function in various species, yet the molecular nature of sleep-memory interaction remains unclear. This article summarizes work that has established the cAMP-PKA-CREB intracellular signaling pathway as a major mechanism in the wakeful consolidation of memory while highlighting newer evidence that this pathway has a role in sleep regulation, in sleep deprivation, and potentially in sleep-memory interactions. It also explores the possibility that sleep might influence memory processing during a sort of molecular replay. The role of new approaches in understanding the nature of sleep-memory interactions is also discussed.

Brain Stimulation During Sleep   85

Lisa Marshall and Jan Born

This article discusses cortical polarization and induction of brain rhythms during sleep via brain electric and magnetic stimulations and resultant functional changes. The studies presented here underscore the strong dependence on the ongoing brain activity of the induced effects on electroencephalogram (EEG) and behavioral measures. The reviewed data on the effect of applied electric currents on brain electric activity and behavior boost the reemerging concept that endogenous oscillating fields are per se of physiologic and functional significance. Applying weak electric currents is a promising approach for investigating different cortical EEG rhythms and their immediate interactions and functional implications for behavior.

Memory, Sleep, and Dreaming: Experiencing Consolidation   97

Erin J. Wamsley and Robert Stickgold

It is now well established that postlearning sleep is beneficial for human memory performance. Learning experiences influence the content of subsequent sleep mentation (ie, dreaming). This article reviews evidence that newly encoded memories are reactivated and consolidated in the sleeping brain, and that this process is directly reflected in the content of concomitant sleep mentation, providing a valuable window into the mnemonic functions of sleep.

The Neurocognitive Effects of Sleep Disruption in Children and Adolescents   109

Louise M. O'Brien

Sleep problems in children and adolescents are common, and sleep disruption is associated with a wide range of behavioral, cognitive, and mood impairments, including hyperactivity, reduced school grades, and depression. Insufficient or fragmented sleep may induce sleepiness, which is associated with problematic behavior, impaired learning, and/or negative mood. Furthermore, treatment of sleep disruption, by improving sleep hygiene or treating specific sleep disorders, is often associated with improvements in daytime performance, suggesting a common mechanism for the behavioral manifestations. This article reviews the daytime manifestations of sleep disruption.

Sleepy Driving   117

Nelson B. Powell and Jason K.M. Chau

Sleepiness and drowsiness are neurophysiologic states that may cause attenuation of vigilance and slowing of reaction times, and thus increase the risks of driving. This article reviews selected peer-reviewed publications from the past and present body of knowledge regarding sleepiness and drowsiness while driving and related accidents, injuries, and possible death. Comparative studies of driving drunk and driving sleepy are reviewed because both exhibit similarly dangerous driving behaviors. It is hoped that some of the information from this article could provide new interest in the necessity of education for sleepy drivers.

Index   125

Foreword

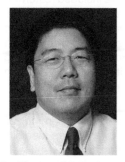

Teofilo Lee-Chiong Jr, MD
Consulting Editor

Given its ubiquity and complexity, it is tempting, and perhaps not unreasonable, to believe that sleep serves a vital physiologic function (ie, it appears unlikely that sleep has no purpose at all). Regrettably, despite advances in techniques of electroencephalography and brain imaging and their application in the study of sleep and waking states, a unitary and comprehensive theory explaining the function of sleep remains elusive. Any theory on the purpose of sleep should account for its function/s in several areas.

FUNCTION ACROSS DIFFERENT SPECIES

Is the function of sleep similar for mammals, birds, reptiles, amphibians, and invertebrates? Are there species of animals that do not sleep at all? Are there differences in the function of sleep between nocturnal versus diurnal species? Do differences in corticocortical wiring between mammals and birds on one hand and reptiles on the other explain the reported variations in expression of sleep and its various stages?

FUNCTION ACROSS GEOLOGIC HISTORY

Why is the human endogenous circadian sleep-wake period (tau) just slightly over, and not exactly, 24 hours in duration? Does tau differ among races, or with aging? Is tau conserved throughout geologic history, being unchanged from its current state in the distant past when the earth "day" was considerably shorter?

FUNCTION ACROSS THE LIFESPAN OF AN INDIVIDUAL

Does sleep serve similar functions in the fetus as it does in the adult? Is preference for "eveningness"

(night owls) or "morningness" (morning larks) that develops among adolescents/younger adults and older adults, respectively, part of the purpose of sleep in these age groups? Are the adverse effects of chronic sleep restriction different for children compared to adults?

FUNCTION IN DIVERSE GEOGRAPHIC AREAS

Is the function of sleep similar for species that live in equatorial versus polar regions? Does the duration of light and darkness that characterize these widely dissimilar locales change the role of sleep during the course of a 12-month period?

FUNCTION OF SPECIFIC SLEEP STAGES

What is the function of non-rapid eye movement (NREM) sleep? What is the function of rapid eye movement (REM) sleep? What of N2 sleep? Or N1 or N3 sleep? Are any of these sleep stages dispensable? Without polysomnography to guide them, can investigators reliably distinguish among the different sleep stages using brain imaging alone?

FUNCTION OF COMPONENTS OF SPECIFIC SLEEP STAGES

Of what use are dreaming, penile tumescence, or rapid eye movements that occur during REM sleep? Would sleep be different if spindles are eliminated? What is the function of a K complex?

FUNCTION OF SLEEP'S EFFECTS ON ORGAN SYSTEMS AND PROCESSES

Finally, do the significant changes in cardiovascular, respiratory, renal, gastrointestinal, metabolic, endocrine, and thermoregulatory physiology that

Sleep Med Clin 6 (2011) xi–xii
doi:10.1016/j.jsmc.2010.12.011

accompany NREM and REM sleep serve any useful function? Would these physiologic processes continue to operate efficiently if sleep is completely abolished? What would happen to memory, executive functions, or inflammatory processes during sleep deprivation?

Several approaches can be employed to investigate the function of sleep. Researchers have compared the physiologic processes that occur during waking and sleep, to identify differences between the two states and to discover if any of them are unique to sleep. Equally instructive are studies on the effects of either sleep deprivation (total or sleep stage-specific) and sleep enhancement on various physiologic processes.

Because it is generally agreed that sleep is generated and maintained by specific neurotransmitters located in specific areas of the brain, researchers have focused their work on the brain. Although theories of sleep function have included restorative and somatic growth, metabolic homeostasis, energy conservation, survival behavior, and immune defense function, the most promising inquiries involve neural growth and processing, neuronal synaptic plasticity, brain development and restoration, learning and memory.

Teofilo Lee-Chiong Jr, MD
Division of Sleep Medicine
National Jewish Health
University of Colorado Denver School of Medicine
1400 Jackson Street, Room J221
Denver, CO 60206, USA

E-mail address:
Lee-ChiongT@NJC.ORG

Preface
Sleep, Learning, and Memory

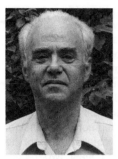

Robert Stickgold, PhD
Guest Editor

Our curiosity over the relationship of sleep to learning and memory has a long history. In the first century AD, the Roman rhetorician Quintilian stated that "the interval of a single night [of sleep] will greatly increase the strength of the memory [as] the power of recollection ... undergoes a process of ripening and maturing,"[1] and the admonition to "sleep on it"—to allow the sleeping brain to process stored information and extract a complex solution for a problem—has been around at least since the 1850s.[2] But scientific investigation of the phenomenon only took off in earnest a century and a half later, in 2000. Since then, research into sleep and memory has grown dramatically, with the number of published papers increasing more than 7-fold from 1999 to 2009 (**Fig. 1**).

Despite this rapid growth, our understanding of sleep's effects on memory remains unclear. Among the most important unanswered questions are (1) the types of memories that undergo processing during sleep (eg, declarative, procedural, classical conditioning, verbal, spatial, motor); (2) the specific memory processes involved (eg, stabilization, enhancement, integration, generalization); (3) the stages of sleep involved with each type of memory and of memory processing; (4) the extent to which the processes occur exclusively, preferentially, or only permissively during sleep; (5) the mechanisms underlying these processes; (6) the phylogenetic and ontogenic variability in these processes; (7) how dreaming interfaces with these processes; and, finally, (8) the impact of this sleep-dependent memory processing on the overall cognitive functioning of the organism.

But as is always true in science, identifying the problem is half the solution, and considerable progress has been made in answering all of these questions. The articles in this issue have been chosen, in part, to address this wide range of questions.

We start with Todd Swick's thorough review of the neurology of sleep. As he aptly notes, "Neurology, by virtue of its study of the brain, is the primary medical science for the elucidation of the anatomy, physiology, pathology, and, ultimately, the function of sleep." All that follows in this issue follows from the neurology he describes.

Swick's article is followed by those by Jessica Payne and by Els van der Helm and Matt Walker, describing, both in broad strokes and in detail, the nature of sleep-dependent memory processing in humans. Payne reviews sleep's facilitation of both perceptual and motor procedural skill learning, and of verbal and spatial, hippocampus-dependent declarative memory, and then moves on to describe more nuanced sleep-dependent transformations of memories that leave them less accurate in their detail, but more ecologically valid and useful. She finishes with a discussion of brain mechanisms that could mediate these effects, providing both neurophysiological and neurochemical evidence for sleep's role in memory processing.

Van der Helm and Walker focus in on sleep and emotions, surveying "an array of diverse findings

Sleep Med Clin 6 (2011) xiii–xv
doi:10.1016/j.jsmc.2010.12.012

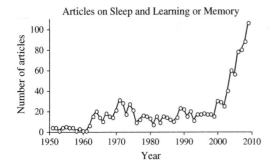

Fig. 1. Publication rates. Number of articles cited in PubMed with MeSH Major Topics of sleep and either learning or memory, by year.

across basic and clinical research domains, resulting in a convergent view of sleep-dependent emotional brain processing." In doing so, they argue for a specific role of sleep in emotional memory processing as well as a more general function in mood regulation that resets the reactivity of limbic and autonomic networks in the brain. Dysregulation of these sleep-dependent processes, they argue, may contribute to a range of mood disturbances.

It is something of an embarrassment that almost all of the studies of sleep and memory reported in the last decade have focused on college-age subjects, although notable forays into both young[3] and elderly[4] populations have been made. In the next article in this issue, Rebecca Gomez and her colleagues review the literature on sleep, learning, and memory in children generally, before turning more specifically to the question of sleep-dependent memory processing in children, convincingly showing that an afternoon nap allows children as young as 15 months of age to extract information about the structure of an artificial grammar to which they were exposed prior to the nap.

The next two articles turn to studies in animals and provide greater insight into the processes and mechanisms of sleep-dependent memory processing. In the first of these, Carlyle Smith reviews the interactions between sleep states and memory processing in rodents, starting with a critical review that supports both the "REM window" hypothesis and the value of sleep deprivation studies. He follows this with a review of studies of hippocampal replay, neurochemical modulation, and genetic manipulation, to provide insights into intracellular mechanisms of sleep-dependent memory processing.

Pepe Hernandez and Ted Abel's thoughtful article juxtaposes molecular mechanisms known to underlie learning and memory consolidation in general with electrophysiological events that are unique to different stages of sleep, describing how these events may serve to modulate the activity of molecular mechanism of learning and consolidation. They finish with a discussion of the methodological problems that must still be addressed before we can comprehensively study sleep-memory interactions at the molecular level.

Our review of mechanisms continues with the article of Lisa Marshall and Jan Born, which looks at the impact of human brain stimulation during sleep on sleep-dependent memory processing. The sleeping brain is not totally resistant to outside influences. Indeed, at least two recent studies have shown that sleep-dependent memory processing can be enhanced by reexposing the sleeping brain to sounds[5] and smells[6] presented during earlier periods of learning. In this article, however, Marshall and Born look at the ability of transcranial magnetic stimulation and direct electrical stimulation, applied to the human brain during sleep, to produce cortical polarization and induce specific EEG rhythms. How these interventions impact on sleep-dependent memory processing provides important insights into the role of specific EEG rhythms in memory processing.

Before turning to the final two articles, we address what is arguably the most obvious, most confusing, and most maligned topic in the field of sleep and memory—dreaming. Here I join with Erin Wamsley to review the literature on this topic. As newly encoded memories are reactivated and consolidated in the sleeping brain, this memory processing is reflected in concomitant dream content. This content, we argue, provides insights into the memory processing functions of sleep that are not available from any other source.

We conclude this issue with two articles that remind the reader that this topic is not merely one of intellectual interest. The impact of poor sleep on the cognitive and behavioral function of all of us, while well known at one level, remains drastically underappreciated at the personal, cultural, medical, and national level. Louise O'Brien, in her review of the neurocognitive deficits seen in children and adolescents with disrupted sleep, and Nelson Powell and Jason Chau, in their article on the impact of sleepiness on driving, remind us of the price paid when we ignore the consequences of poor sleep. They also remind us how much remains to be discovered on this critical topic. In many ways, the measure of this issue's success should not be how well it reviews what is known about sleep, memory, and learning, but by how effectively it inspires you, the reader, to take what you learn here, raise new questions, and then go out and answer them. Bon voyage!

Robert Stickgold, PhD
Department of Psychiatry
Beth Israel Deaconess Medical Center
330 Brookline Avenue, E/FD 861
Boston, MA 02215, USA

E-mail address:
rstickgold@hms.harvard.edu

REFERENCES

1. Quintilian, The institutio oratoria of Quintilian. Translated by HE Butler, Butler HE, editor. Cambridge: Harvard University Press; 1920. Book XI, II, 43–4.

2. Dickens C. Hard Times. Household Words. Wkly J 1854;IX(213):214.

3. Backhaus J, Hoeckesfeld R, Born J, et al. Immediate as well as delayed post learning sleep but not wakefulness enhances declarative memory consolidation in children. Neurobiol Learn Mem 2008;89(1): 76–80.

4. Spencer RM, Gouw AM, Ivry RB. Age-related decline of sleep-dependent consolidation. Learn Mem 2007; 14(7):480–4.

5. Rudoy JD, Voss JL, Westerberg CE, et al. Strengthening individual memories by reactivating them during sleep. Science 2009;326(5956):1079.

6. Rasch B, Büchel C, Gais S, et al. Odor cues during slow-wave sleep prompt declarative memory consolidation. Science 2007;315(5817):1426–9.

The Neurology of Sleep

Todd J. Swick, MD[a,b,*]

KEYWORDS

- Acetylcholine • Serotonin • Dopamine • Norepinephrine
- Histamine • Orexin • Melatonin • Circadian rhythm

Neurology, by virtue of its study of the brain, is the primary medical science for the elucidation of the anatomy, physiology, pathology, and, ultimately, the function of sleep.

HISTORICAL CONTEXT

The Greco-Roman concepts of sleep were based on their belief that there were gods and goddesses that controlled the minor and major events of their lives. They identified the goddess of night (Nyx) who had two sons: Hypnos (the god of sleep) and his brother, Thanantos (the god of death). Hypnos sprinkled drops of poppy milk into people's eyes so that the opium would make them fall asleep and then fanned sleeping persons with his wings to enable them to sleep in comfort. As late as the beginning of the Common Era, Ovid wrote that Hypnos lived with his "thousand children," the Dreams, in a cave in the Caucasus. The river of Lethe (the river of forgetfulness) was believed to run through this cave.[1]

In ancient Greece, if citizens were unable to sleep because of their problems, they visited one of the many sanitariums dedicated to Asclepios (the Greek god of medicine), where the afflicted spent 3 weeks in rest, thought, and meditation, soothed by gentle music, and then, having their balance restored, would be able to sleep again (obviously predating the concept of managed care).[2]

From the time of the Middle Ages until the Renaissance, there were discrete changes in the concept of sleep. More concrete explanations of sleep were enunciated by Lucretius, the Epicurean poet and philosopher, when he described "sleep as the absence of wakefulness".[3] This was the prevailing view through the centuries. As medical science advanced with the discovery of the circulatory system and as the young field of neurology was explored, there was renewed interest in the science of sleep and wakefulness.

In 1866, the Surgeon General of the United States, William A. Hammond, wrote a treatise, "On Wakefulness: With an Introductory Chapter on the Physiology of Sleep," arguing against the prevailing opinion of his day that sleep began as a consequence of "congestion of the cerebral vessels." He pointed out several observations that were quoted in contemporary textbooks of medical physiology of his time: (1) stupor never occurs in healthy individuals, whereas sleep is a necessity of life; (2) it is easy to awaken a person from sleep, whereas it often is impossible to arouse him from stupor; (3) in sleep the mind is active and in stupor it is as if it were dead; and (4) congestion of cerebral vessels causes stupor, not sleep. He quotes another nineteenth-century physician, Dr Arthur Durham: "During sleep, the brain is in a comparatively bloodless condition and the blood in the encephalic vessels is not only diminished in quantity but moves with diminished rapidity. Whatever increases the activity of the cerebral circulation tends to preserve wakefulness and whatever decreases the activity of the cerebral circulation and, at the same time, is not inconsistent with the general health of the body tends to induce and favor sleep".[4]

Although still surrounded by myth and less than perfect science, the concept of the neural control of sleep was established. From 1916 through

This article originally appeared in the November 2005 issue of *Neurologic Clinics of North America* 23:4.
[a] School of Medicine, University of Texas-Houston, Houston, TX, USA
[b] The Houston Sleep Center, Houston, TX, USA
* University of Texas-Houston, 7500 San Felipe, Suite 525, Houston, TX 77063.
E-mail address: tswick@houstonsleepcenter.com

Sleep Med Clin 6 (2011) 1–14
doi:10.1016/j.jsmc.2010.12.009

1928, the world was ravaged by an epidemic of influenza with tens of thousands of deaths, the victims sustaining many neurologic signs and symptoms. During the acute phase of the illness, some patients exhibited severe insomnia and many more exhibited severe hypersomnia, whereas many survivors exhibited signs of Parkinsonism.

In 1917, von Economo published his first paper on encephalitis lethargica and on December 3, 1929, he read a paper before the College of Physicians and Surgeons of Columbia University in New York City entitled, "Sleep as a Problem of Localization." He stated that patients who had insomnia had lesions in the anterior portion of their hypothalamus and that patients who had hypersomnia had lesions in the posterior aspect of the hypothalamus. He designated this area of the "interbrain" as the "center for regulation of sleep." Thus, the prevailing concept espoused by such luminaries as Lhermitte and Dejerine that "sleep cannot be localized" was put to rest.[5,6]

In 1928, Berger demonstrated that the brain produced clearly identifiable electrical activity that could be recorded using surface electrodes and that there existed a different pattern of electrical activity of the brain during consciousness compared with sleep.[6,7]

In 1935, Bremer reported on the effects of transection of the brainstem of cats at the pontine-midbrain level (cerveau isolé) versus transection at the medullary-spinal cord level (encéphale isolé). He found that the cerveau isolé animals maintained a continuous sleep-like state with synchronous slow wave activity, whereas the encéphale isolé cats looked awake and their electroencephalograms (EEGs) contained synchronous and de-synchronized activity resembling sleep-wake cycling. Bremer went on to hypothesize that sleep was a passive process and that wakefulness required a high level of continuous sensory input from the periphery to maintain activity within the cerebral hemispheres.[8]

Bremer's work rekindled research concerning the observations of y Cajal and Papez. In 1909 y Cajal described an extensive network of neurons that ascended and descended through the brainstem. This was refined further by observations of Papez who in 1926 published a more complete description of the reticular formation and its caudal projections down into the spinal cord in cats.[9,10]

In 1942, Morison and Dempsey published a series of articles that described a diffuse "nonspecific" thalamocortical recruiting system. They differentiated this "nonspecific" system from the primary sensory input (ie, "specific" system [described by Lorente de No in 1938], acting through direct thalamic relays).[11,12]

In 1949, Moruzzi and Magoun identified the ascending reticular activating system "whose direct stimulation activates or desynchronizes the EEG, replacing high-voltage slow waves with low-voltage fast activity." They went on to state, "the effect is exerted generally upon the cortex and is mediated, in part, at least, by the diffuse thalamic projection system".[13]

By the middle of the twentieth century it was established that sleep and wakefulness were different states that are controlled by the brain and that sleep was not a passive period of time devoid of activity. Jouvet and colleagues described more precise localizations of the neural loci of sleep and its constituents where results of lesion studies demonstrated that the brainstem contains the site of rapid eye movement (REM) sleep neural activity. Transections of a cat brain at a level just above the midbrain-pons junction preserved the appearance of REM-sleep activity, whereas transections in the pons abolished the appearance of REM sleep.[14–16]

With the discoveries of REM and non-REM (NREM) sleep by Aserinsky and Kleitman and REM/NREM cycling by Dement and Kleitman, the door finally was opened for researchers to gain more exact insights into the study of the science of sleep and wakefulness.[17–19]

SLEEP AND WAKE STATES

People exist in one of three behavioral states during normal functioning: (1) wakefulness; (2) NREM sleep; and (3) REM sleep (**Fig. 1**). These states are characterized by specific changes in EEG, eye movements, and muscle activity. Wakefulness is characterized by well-recognized patterns on surface EEG recording. Alpha activity (8–12 Hz waves of <50 μV amplitude) occurs when individuals are resting with their eyes closed. The rhythms are most evident in the parieto-occipital areas of the head. Alpha rhythm is attenuated or blocked by attention, especially visual (eye-opening) and mental effort. Eye movements are purposeful and conjugate. Muscle tone is variable but never absent.

The transition to and from sleep is not an all-or-none phenomenon but a continuum. Criteria are set (Rechtschaffen and Kales), however, that allow for the clinical and research separation of individual sleep states in a reproducible fashion.[20] Early drowsiness can be produced by boredom or fatigue and is characterized by EEG changes of gradual or rapid "alpha dropout." Theta range rhythms appear (4.5–7.5 Hz) and can be mixed with low-voltage 15- to 25-Hz activity. Deepening of drowsiness is characterized by increasing slow activity with transients of 2 to 4 Hz and 4.5

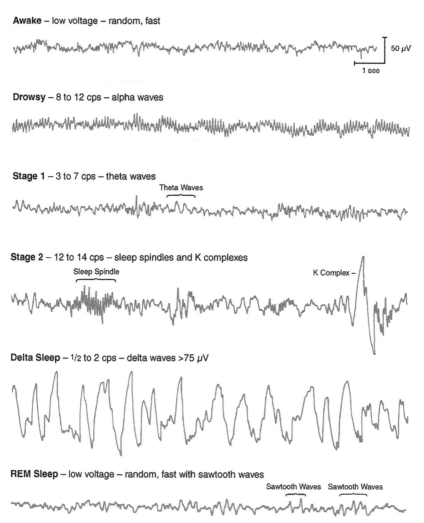

Fig. 1. EEG patterns from wakefulness into drowsiness and then into stages 1 through 4 NREM sleep and into REM sleep. Sleep spindles and K complexes are noted in stage 2 sleep and saw-tooth waves are seen in REM sleep. (*Adapted from* Hauri P. The sleep disorders. Curr Concepts 1982;7; with permission.)

to 7 Hz. The hallmark of deep drowsiness is the appearance of vertex sharp waves that can appear as isolated events or can occur in trains of events. Accompanying the slowing of the background rhythm is the appearance of slow-rolling eye movements and moderately elevated muscle tone.

It has been stated that the first "unequivocal" stage of sleep is stage 2. This stage is characterized by the presence of sleep spindles that have a frequency of 12 to 14 Hz with progressively increasing and then progressively decreasing amplitude lasting 0.5 to 2 seconds in duration. Sleep spindles are believed to arise from generators located in the reticular nucleus of the thalamus and begin to appear as brainstem nuclei, particularly the cholinergic neurons, diminish their firing rates.[21] It is believed that sleep spindles represent the electrical signature of cerebral deafferentation

that occurs when primary sensory pathways are gated.

The second hallmark of stage 2 sleep is the appearance of K complexes. These are evoked cortical responses to arousing stimuli and are characterized by a sharp negative wave followed by a slower positive wave with a minimum duration of 0.5 seconds. Slow eye movements persist generally for only a brief time after the appearance of sleep spindles and K complexes and the electromyogram shows persistence of moderate muscle tone.[22]

Deep sleep, also known as slow wave sleep (SWS), comprises stage 3 and stage 4 in the Rechtschaffen and Kales criteria. Here, the background rhythm is at its slowest frequency of the sleep period (in the range of 0.5–3 Hz) with an amplitude of greater than 75 μV. Eye movements are absent and the electromyogram tone remains elevated but less than stages 1 and 2 (**Fig. 2**). Stage 3 is defined as delta activity comprising less than 50% of a recording epoch (30 seconds) and stage 4 represents greater than 50% in delta frequencies. The overall pattern of the EEG is one of high voltage synchronous slow wave activity seen over the entire brain. Cortical cells that are governed by cells in the dorsal thalamus and transmitted via the vast array of the thalamocortical projections generate these waves. As the dorsal and reticulothalamic nuclei become more hyperpolarized, sleep spindles diminish and slower delta waves increase. The appearance of the very low frequency slow-waves marks the virtual cessation of firing of the cholinergic neurons in the brainstem.

REM sleep, or paradoxic sleep, represents the time of cortical activation as evidenced by a rapid transition to a higher frequency rhythm of the EEG (rapid, low-voltage, irregular activity). REMs occur in phasic bursts and there is the occurrence of large burst potentials that originate in the pons and pass rapidly to the lateral geniculate body and then to the occipital lobe (**P**ons **G**eniculate **O**ccipital-waves).[23] There is a marked reduction in skeletal muscle tone except for the diaphragm and the extraocular eye muscles by way of activation of the medial medulla, which inhibits motor neurons by the release of glycine onto spinal and brainstem neurons producing hyperpolarization and inhibition.

ASCENDING RETICULAR SYSTEM

As discussed previously, Moruzzi and Magoun identified the activating system as having a significant role in the maintenance of wakefulness and its EEG correlates.[13] The neurons of the reticular activating system receive input from a range of neural networks, including visceral, somatic, and special sensory systems. The inputs travel through two pathways, a dorsal pathway to the thalamic nuclei and a ventral pathway to the hypothalamus. The neurotransmitters include acetylcholine, serotonin, noradrenalin, dopamine, histamine, and Hypocretin (Orexin) (**Figs. 3** and **4**).

Acetylcholine

Steriade and colleages identified groups of cells in the pons-midbrain junction projecting to the thalamus that increased their firing rate approximately a minute before the first change to a desynchronized state was noted on the EEG.[24] These cell groups later were identified as the laterodorsal tegmental (LDT) and pedunculopontine tegmental (PPT) nuclei that contained acetylcholine as their neurotransmitter. These cholinergic neurons send fibers via the dorsal pathway to the thalamus where they project specifically to the intralaminar nuclei, the thalamic relay nuclei, and the reticular nucleus. When active, the cholinergic projections allow flow of information through the thalamus, to and from the cerebral cortex, and promote cortical desynchronization (thalamocortical activation). The activity of the LDT-PPT neurons changes with the appearance of each of the states of sleep and wakefulness. During wakefulness, the neurons fire rapidly. With the onset of stage 1 and 2 of NREM sleep, the LDT-PPT neurons slow their firing rate and in SWS the neurons become quiet. During

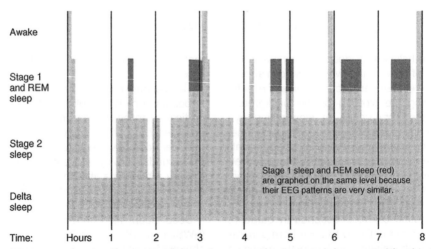

Fig. 2. Sleep hypnogram showing the course of sleep stages over the nocturnal sleep period for this young (ages 20–30) adult. Note the rapid descent into SWS (delta sleep) at the beginning of the nights and the 90-minute cycling of REM sleep. Note that most of SWS, or delta sleep, takes place in the first half of the night and REM sleep increases in period length as the night progresses, with the longest REM episode occurring just before sleep offset. (*Adapted from* Hauri P. The sleep disorders. Curr Concepts 1982;8; with permission.)

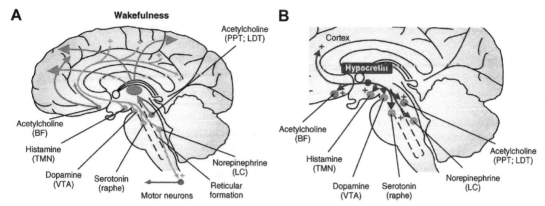

Fig. 3. (*A*) Dorsal and ventral reticular formations are shown with the dorsal cholinergic system (*blue*) sending fibers into the thalamus (*green*) and basal forebrain. The thalamus then projects out over the entire cortex by way of the thalamocortical projections. The ventral aminergic pathway is associated with wakefulness. (*B*) The hypocretin cell group in the lateral and posterior hypothalamus sends excitatory neurons to the cholinergic and monoaminergic groups of the reticular formation (all awake-promoting cell groups). (*Adapted from* España R, Scammell TE. Sleep neurobiology for the clinician. Sleep 2004;27:811–20; with permission.)

REM sleep, their activity suddenly becomes active again when they are released from monoamine-mediated inhibition.[25–28]

There also are cholinergic neurons in the basal forebrain (magnocellular fields in the basal nucleus of Meynert). These neurons send projections throughout the cortex, hippocampus, and amygdala. Firing rates are highest during wakefulness and REM sleep and are lowest during NREM sleep.[29]

Monoaminergic Systems

The second branch of the reticular activating system is the branch that innervates the hypothalamus via the ventral route. The neurons that make up these fibers are monoaminergic and include

the noradrenergic locus coeruleus (LC), the serotoninergic dorsal raphe and median raphe nuclei, and dopaminergic cells in the periaqueductal gray.[30,31] These fibers are joined by fibers from the histaminergic neurons originating in the tuberomammillary nucleus (TMN),[32,33] hypocretin (orexin) input from the lateral hypothalamus, melatonin-concentrating hormone-containing neurons, and the basal forebrain cholinergic nuclei.[34–40] These then send fibers back to the basal forebrain, the ventral preoptic area, and, subsequently, the entire cerebral cortex.

Like the cholinergic LDT-PPT neurons, the monoaminergic neurons—noradrenergic LC, serotonergic raphe, and histaminergic (TMN)—also have a state-specific firing rate. These collectively fire fastest during wakefulness, slow down during NREM sleep, and nearly stop firing during REM

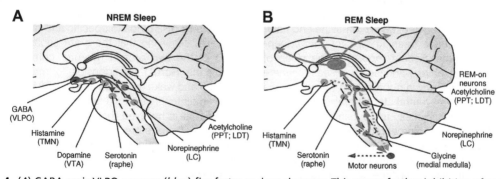

Fig. 4. (*A*) GABA-ergic VLPO neurons (*blue*) fire faster as sleep deepens. This causes further inhibition of arousal centers in LDT-PPT and the monoaminergic brainstem groups TMN, ventral tegmental area (VTA), the raphe, and the LC. (*B*) REM-on cells in LDT-PPT are disinhibited by GABA-ergic cells also in the LDT-PPT. This causes activation of the thalamorcortical pathways producing cortical desynchronization. There are efferents to the medial medulla from the SLD (subcoeruleus area), which they synapse on GABA-ergic and glycinergic neruons to produce inhibition of motor nuerons in the brainstem and spinal cord to produce muscle atonia. (*Adapted from* España R, Scammell TE. Sleep neurobiology for the clinician. Sleep 2004;27:811–20; with permission.)

sleep.[28] The specific monoamines are associated with the maintenance of wakefulness.

Norepinephrine and Histamine

Norepinephrine (NE) is released during wakefulness,[41] and pharmacologic manipulation with NE or NE agonist drugs uniformly produces an increase in waking behavior and exhibits inhibitory mechanisms on sleep production. Likewise, histamine is believed to be the "master" wakefulness-promoting neurotransmitter, with high activity during wakefulness and decreasing activity during NREM sleep down to its lowest levels during REM sleep. It is well known that histamine blockers promote sleep onset and increase NREM sleep.[42] Recent studies investigating H_3 receptor agonists suggest that these moieties stimulate autoinhibitory receptors on histamine and other aminergic neurons and produce augmentation of sleep onset.[43]

Serotonin

The physiologic effects of serotonin on sleep and wake behavior is controversial, with conflicting reports that serotonin promotes sleep and induces wakefulness. Most recent evidence, however, shows that serotonin promotes wakefulness with an increase in sleep-onset latency and a decrease in REM sleep. Clinically, down-regulation of serotonin signaling may be the cause of hypersomnia seen when selective serotinin reuptake inhibitors first are initiated in depressed patients.[44,45]

Dopamine

Dopamine (DA) and its role in sleep-wake regulation remain unclear. From a pharmacologic standpoint, the release of DA and its reuptake inhibition by powerful stimulants, such as amphetamines, shows its wakefulness-promoting properties.[46–48] Dopamine blockers (eg, chlorpromazine and haloperidol) long have been known for their sleep-inducing effects. Recent reports of the sleep of patients who have Parkinson's disease, where there is a deficiency in dopamine in the substantia nigra and the ventral tegmental area, show remarkable similarities to patients who have narcolepsy (ie, fragmented nocturnal sleep), early-onset REM periods, REM sleep behavior disorder, and multiple sleep latency test, demonstrating pathologic daytime sleepiness with an increase in sleep-onset REM periods.[47] The confound is that some patients (those who have Parkinson's disease and those who are being treated with DA receptor agonists for restless legs syndrome) on occasion experience sudden sleep attacks. One possible explanation for this incongruity is that low doses of DA receptor agonists bind to autoinhibitory receptors on DA neurons, further decreasing DA signaling and thus decreasing the wakefulness drive.[49]

Hypocretin (orexin)

The recent discovery of excitatory sleep-wake neuropeptides hypocretin (HcrtR1 and HcrtR2), also known as orexin (orexin-1 and orexin-2), has added significant insight into the regulation of the sleep-wake state and offered explanations as to the cause of narcolepsy.[50–53] These neuropeptides are produced by a small cluster of neurons in the lateral, posterior, and perifornical areas of the hypothalamus that have diffuse projections throughout the central nervous system.[34] These areas of the hypothalamus receive dense input from the monoaminergic and cholinergic brainstem nuclei. The neurons of the hypocretin producing cell groups are most active during waking, particularly during periods of increased psychomotor activity, and significantly decrease in firing during NREM and REM sleep.[28]

More than 90% of narcoleptics who have cataplexy have low or undetectable levels of hypocretin in their cerebrospinal fluid, and postmortem analysis of brains of patients who have narcolepsy show a marked reduction in the number of hypocretin neurons.[52,53] The hypocretin neurons are activated by glutamate that in turn increases the amount of glutamate in the surrounding cells of the hypothalamus that creates a positive feedback system to sustain the firing of the hypocretin neurons.

Recent studies suggest that the two hypocretin moieties, HcrtR1 and HcrtR2, perform distinct functions in terms of modulation of sleep and its constituent parts. Although both mediate excitatory responses, HcrtR1 binds to specific G-proteins, whereas HcrtR2 binds to specific and nonspecific proteins, signifying that there are separate functions of the two protein receptor complexes. It seems that HcrtR1 is responsible for maintenance of sleep and wake episodes and HcrtR2 is involved in the maintenance of skeletal muscle tone while awake.[54] It is believed that hypocretin deficiency leads to sleep state instability with increased numbers of transitions between sleep and wakefulness and between REM sleep phenomena and wakefulness.

The understanding of the orchestration of the timing of sleep onset and then the initiation of the ultradian rhythm of REM and NREM sleep is the Holy Grail of sleep research. Von Economo hypothesizes that within the hypothalamus there are two distinct sites, one that promotes wakefulness and a second that promotes sleep.[5] Recent findings confirm his theories and offer a better understanding of the sleep-onset and maintenance mechanisms.

By identifying modulators of the histaminergic neurons of the TMN, Sherin and coworkers show that γ-aminobutyric acid (GABA)-ergic inputs that originate in the ventrolateral preoptic (VLPO) area and the extended VLPO area of the hypothalamus inhibit the TMN.[55] There also is further inhibitory input to the TMN from fibers that have their cell bodies scattered more diffusely in the lateral hypothalamus (the extended VLPO). In addition to GABA, these neurons contain the inhibitory neuropeptide, galanin.[25] There also are inhibitory efferents to other monoaminergic nuclei, such as the raphe nuclei and the LC. Thus, by inhibiting the wake promoting action of these monoaminergic amines, the VLPO promotes the onset of sleep. Alternatively, these same monoaminergic cell groups also supply efferents back to the VLPO. There also is input from hypocretin-containing cells in the dorsolateral hypothalamus. This reciprocal innervation sets the stage for control of the sleep-wake switch. In addition, known sleep-inducing substances (somnogens), such as adenosine, increase activity in the VLPO, in turn promoting sleep, allowing more modulatory input to the sleep-wake control.[56–59] This scenario has led to the hypothesis that there is a bistable sleep-wake switch, where the VLPO and arousal systems are inhibited reciprocally.[60]

The firing rates of VLPO neurons increase during sleep and get progressively faster as sleep deepens (SWS). This increased firing causes further inhibition of arousal centers that allow less interrupted and thereby deeper sleep. In the opposite scenario, wakefulness causes inhibition of the VLPO that ensures full wakefulness without letting drowsiness cause diminished cognitive abilities. Saper and coworkers describe this as a sleep-wake "flip-flop" switch, with each half of the mechanism strongly inhibiting the other. Full change of state requires overwhelming forces, such as accumulated homeostatic sleep drive, coupled with the appropriate circadian influence to drive the switch into its opposite configuration.[60]

This model can explain how the behavioral states of wakefulness and sleep can transition from one to the other and maintain the state regardless of constantly changing homeostatic forces that accumulate and dissipate over the course of a day, allowing the circadian influences to ensure 24-hour rhythmicity.

Once sleep onset occurs, a second set of neuronal interactions occur that account for NREM/REM cycling. Firing of VLPO neurons increases as sleep gets deeper. A transition occurs during NREM sleep when GABA-ergic LPT neurons disinhibit REM-on neurons located in and near the cholinergic neural group of the LDT-PPT. Acetylcholine is released into the thalamus, producing cortical desynchrony.[61,62] The aminergic neurons of the TMN, raphe, and LC fall silent (most likely mediated through afferents in the area of the extended VLPO) (**Fig. 5, Table 1**).[28]

REM sleep can be dissociated into its different components, including muscle atonia, EEG desynchronization, PGO waves, and REMs. Each of these clinical manifestations of REM sleep is under the control of discrete cell groups within the pontine reticular formation and the midbrain reticular formation, which includes the sublateral dorsal area (SLD), also known as the subcoeruleus area. These cell groups are called effector neurons.[64] These cell groups are silent during NREM sleep. They begin to depolarize 30 to 60 seconds before the first sign of REM sleep occurs, the PGO waves. The pontine

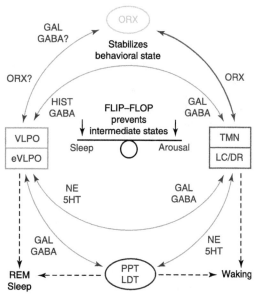

Fig. 5. The two main centers for sleep and arousal are shown. The VLPO and the extended VLPO (eVLPO) are the centers for sleep maintenance, whereas the TMN, LC, and dorsal raphe (DR) are all monoaminergic wakefulness-promoting neural groups. The inhibitory pathways are in red and the excitatory pathways are in green. Orexin/hypocretin shown at the top stabilizes the two states and prevents rapid cycling. During wakefulness there is inhibition of the VLPO and eVLPO, and during sleep there is inhibition of the monoaminergic stimulatory cell groups. (*From* Saper CB, Chou TC, Scammell TE. The sleep switch: hypothalamic control of sleep and wakefulness. Trends Neurosci 2001;24:729.)

Table 1
State-specific firing rates of brainstem and cortical neuronal groups

Site	Neurotransmitter	Wakefulness	Non–rapid Eye Movement Sleep	Rapid Eye Movement Sleep
Basal forebrain	Acetylcholine	++++	+	++++
Laterodorsol tegmentum/ pedunculopontine tegementum	Acetylcholine	++++	+++ → 0	++++
Dorsal and median raphe	Serotonin	++++	++	0
Loceus coerulus	NE	++++	++	0
Tuberomammillary nucleus	Histamine	++++	++	0
Posterior/lateral hypothalamus	Hypocretin/orexin	++++	+	+
Ventrolateral preoptic area	GABA	+	+++	++++

reticular formation/midbrain reticular formation then undergoes further neuronal depolarization, leading to the development of action potentials in these cell groups. The action potentials increase as REM sleep starts and this high rate of firing is maintained throughout the REM sleep episode.

SLD neurons project to the ventrolateral medulla and the spinal cord, where they synapse on GABA-ergic and glycinergic neurons to produce hyperpolarization and inhibition of motor neurons in the brainstem and spinal cord, thus accounting for the widespread muscle atonia of REM sleep. The medial medulla inhibits motor neurons further by reducing excitatory output from the LC and red nucleus.[63,66] Lesions of the SLD cause REM without atonia.[65]

Neurons in the midbrain reticular formation are important in mediating EEG desynchronization characterized by low-voltage, fast-frequency EEG.

The SLD also contains GABA-ergic efferents that feed back and can inhibit the LPT. This mutual inhibition between the LPT and SLD creates another flip-flop switch that can explain the ultradian rhythm of NREM and REM; however, this makes the REM/NREM cycling vulnerable to extrinsic perturbations. It is believed that hypocretin neurons prevent unwanted transitions by weighing in on the REM-off side during wakefulness. This can explain the intrusion of REM sleep components into wakefulness that is characteristic of narcolepsy, where lack of hypocretin signaling allows the SLD and LDT to transition independently into atonia (cataplexy) and REM forebrain phenomena (LDT causes hypnagogic hallucinations).[65]

CIRCADIAN RHYTHM
Suprachiasmatic Nucleus

Circadian rhythms are biologic activities that recur approximately every 24 hours. In the absence of external timing cues (zeitgebers), some of these processes remain rhythmic (ie, "run free") with an approximately 24-hour period. In mammals, the suprachiasmatic nucleus (SCN) is the pacemaker for maintaining circadian sleep-wake cycles, body temperature changes, hormonal releases, and cyclic behavioral patterns. The SCN is located in the ventromedial hypothalamus immediately dorsal to the optic chiasm.

In mammals, the most important stimulus for the time-locked regulation of the circadian rhythm is light. The SCN has a direct afferent connection from the retina via the retinohypothalamic tract.[67] Activation is via a unique class of melanopsin-containing photopigment cells in the retinal ganglia providing the main input for photic entrainment. The putative neurotransmitter in the retinohypothalamic tract is the excitatory amino acid, glutamate.[68]

Nonphotic entrainment remains controversial. It generally is believed that nonphotic input to the SCN is mediated by thalamic input under the influence of serotoninergic neurons.[69] There also are, however, afferents from the histaminergic TMS and cholinergic inputs from multiple forebrain and brainstem regions, in particular the pedunculopontine tegmentum.[70]

There are diffuse projections from the paraventricular nucleus of the thalamus and inputs from the hypothalamus itself, via the geniculohypothalamic tract (GHT). It is believed that input from the GHT is critical in nonphotic entrainment. The GHT originates from cells in the intergeniculate leaflet (IGL), which is located between the dorsal and ventrolateral geniculate nuclei in the thalamus.[71] The IGL has inputs from the retina, the noradrenergic LC, and the serotonergic raphe.[72] Efferents project to the contralateral IGL, the SCN and the peri-SCN area, the pineal, the accessory optic system the superior colliculus, the zona incerta, and the pretectum.

Besides glutamate, other neurotransmitters associated with the SCN include GABA, vasoactive intestinal protein, neuropeptide Y (NPY), met-enkephalin and orphanin-FQ.[73] NPY phase shifts circadian rhythms. Injecting antiserum to NPY into the SCN area can block its effect. Serotonin input from the median raphe nucleus goes directly into the SCN. Serotonergic input from the dorsal raphe, however, comes via projections to the IGL that then feed into the SCN via NPY.[74]

Efferents from the SCN project to four main areas. One group of fibers goes dorsally to the paraventricular area of the thalamus and the posterior hypothalamus. A second group of efferents goes to nuclei located rostral to the SCN, in particular, the medial preoptic area. The third group of fibers runs caudally from the SCN to the anterior, medial, and lateral hypothalamic areas. The fourth group of fibers runs dorsal to the optic tracts into the ventrolateral geniculate nucleus. Thus, there are extensive innervations from the SCN back into the hypothalamus and thalamus to control a complex series of interactions involving hormonal, behavioral, and temperature control.[75]

Clock Genes

The neurons within the SCN generate the circadian rhythm by means of oscillatory protein synthesis via several clock genes. The first gene, *Period* (*Per*), which encodes a clock component protein, PER, was discovered in 1971.[76] Since then, at least eight genes have been identified that are involved with mammalian clock regulation. There are three *Period* genes (*mPer1, mPer2,* and *mPer3*), two *Cryptochrome* genes (*mCry1* and *mCry2*), *Clock* gene, *Bmal 1* or *Mop3*, and *Cklε*.[76] Through a series of experiments that looked at mutations of these clock genes and the resultant physiologic and behavioral changes that they produced, Daan and colleagues propose a model that explains the negative feedback control that produces the 24-hour rhythms and allows for adjustment to seasonal changes in the change in the length of daylight with a morning oscillator (M) that phase advances the circadian rhythm by sensing light at dawn and an evening oscillator

(E) that phase delays the rhythm keyed to decreasing light at dusk.[78]

Within the nucleus of a SCN neuron, the CLOCK and BMAL1 proteins form a heterodimer that binds to the promoters of the *Per1* and *Per2* genes that activate their transcription. The PER1 and PER2 proteins, after phosphylation in the cytoplasm, interact with clock gene products, CRY1 and CRY2 proteins. These *Cry* genes have opposite effects of the *Per1* and *Per2* genes. It also is observed that *Per1* (M) and *Per2* (E) gene expression have different light responsiveness. Thus, the clock can be seen as an oscillator that is stabilized by two regulatory loops. The first is the M that is sensitive to dawn and the reappearance of sunlight. The second is an E tracking the fading of light. After the modulation by the CRY1 proteins, the PER1/CRY1 heterodime is transported back into the nucleus and turns off the transcription of CLOCK/BMAL1, thereby inhibiting *Per1* and *Cry1* transcription. Likewise, the PER2/CRY2 heterodime regulates *Per2* and *Cry2* transcription.[77]

HOMESTATIC AND CIRCADIAN SLEEP-WAKE INTERACTIONS

Experimental studies show that in addition to the circadian timing mechanism, there is a second force that also regulates the sleep-wake cycle, known as the homeostatic sleep process. Well before the SCN was identified as the "master clock," the main theories of why humans sleep had to do with maintenance of physiologic equilibrium (homeostasis).[79]

In 1910, Legendre and Pieron found that the cerebrospinal fluid of sleep-deprived dogs induced sleep in dogs with no loss of sleep when injected into their ventricular system. The idea that there is a toxin or toxic byproduct or other sleep factor that builds up when there is sleep loss or accumulates after repeated bouts of insufficient sleep was established.[80]

There is evidence that adenosine may be the sleep-inducing factor, or somnogen. Adenosine levels in the basal forebrain rise with sleep deprivation and fall rapidly during the subsequent sleep period. This may explain why caffeine, an adenosine A1 receptor blocker, is able to maintain alertness. It seems that adenosine promotes sleep by direct inhibition of wake-promoting neural groups and by disinhibiting the sleep-promoting VLPO neurons.[56]

Adenosine may not be the only somnogen present. Infectious processes can induce sleep. Sleep also is induced by cytokines, such as interleukin-1β, tumor necrosis factor α, and interferon-α.[81] Cytokines also induce the production of prostaglandin D2 that promotes REM and NREM sleep.

To better understand the interaction of the two processes, several experimental paradigms were developed. One set of experiments involved sleep-deprivation studies, in which sleep was eliminated completely for extended periods of time. Even though the overall "sleep pressure" increased, there was still was a discernable 24-hour cycle, with increased sleep propensity during what ordinarily is the subject's nighttime and increased alertness during the subject's day.[82] Several studies demonstrate that there are actually two times of increased sleep propensity, one less robust period during the early afternoon and a second more powerful period at night. All studies show the greatest increase in sleepiness occurs in the early morning hours, whereas the least sleepiness occurs in the early evening.[83]

A second set of experiments involved sleep displacement, where sleep-onset times were shifted. When sleep was shifted by 12 hours, there was a significant increase in wakefulness in the beginning of the sleep period accompanied by a shift of REM sleep to the first third to half of the night (REM sleep normally is maximal during the second half of the night). Thus, there was a decrease in the first REM latency and an increase in wakefulness after sleep onset.[84] This corresponds to the clinical issue of shift workers, who, after working at night, report fragmented and nonrestorative sleep when their rest cycle takes place during the day.

Some of the earliest work involved temporal isolation studies, where subjects were placed in environments where there were no discernable cues to the external environment (ie, all time cues [zeitgebers] were removed). The findings showed that the sleep-wake cycle tended to increase to somewhat less than 25 hours and the diurnal temperature curve followed suit. This was called a free-running rhythm.[85]

The sleep-wake cycle is synchronized with the ambient light-dark cycle, with the peak rectal temperature occurring in the late afternoon to early evening. The nadir occurs in the second half of the sleep period. After several days in a free-running environment, however, the temperature peak advances to the first half of the activity period and the nadir changes to the first half of the sleep period. In subjects whose sleep onset occurred close to their temperature minimum, sleep offset took place on the rising limb of the temperature cycle. The total amount of sleep was reduced even when the "sleep pressure" was increasing, as measured by the total amount of prior wakefulness.

Another significant observation of these temporal isolation subjects was that many of them exhibited a spontaneous dissociation of their temperature cycles from their rest-activity cycles after several days. This is called internal desynchronization.

Zulley found that in internally desynchronized subjects, the circadian temperature curve influenced not only the duration of sleep but also the propensity of falling asleep.[86] Czeisler and coworkers show that the timing of REM sleep is dependent on the circadian phase of the temperature cycle at sleep onset and not on the amount of prior wakefulness. Further studies show that there are two "zones" of high probability for going to sleep and two "zones" of a low probability of falling asleep.[87]

These findings led to what appeared to be a paradoxic conclusion (ie, it is most difficult to fall asleep shortly before what for most people is their regular bedtime). The two zones of highest sleep propensity were analyzed further using nap times in internally desynchronized subjects. Zulley and Campbell found that naps clustered at two circadian phases, one at the temperature nadir and a second at a point halfway between two successive temperature nadirs. They explained this by the existence not only of a primary sleep period but also a secondary circadian sleep period that, under normally entrained conditions, corresponds to the early afternoon.[88]

FORCED DESYNCHRONY

Another experimental paradigm used a forced day length close to, but not exactly, that of a 24-hour time period (eg, 22.7 or 25.3 hours). The duration of wakefulness between successive sleep periods remained constant, but sleep onset occurred at different circadian phases. The net effect was to allow the body temperature rhythm to run free and to separate the circadian dependent processes from the homeostatic processes.

Using the forced desynchrony protocol, it was established that the human circadian clock is much closer to the environmental diurnal day-night cycle (24 hours ± 10 minutes) and it is the same in all age groups. Thus, the concept that aging brings on circadian changes was challenged successfully.[89]

Sleep pressure, as measured by sleep-onset latency, is maximal near the nadir of core body temperature that is close to the usual wake time in normally entrained conditions. The drive to maintain wakefulness is strongest during the evening hours near the temperature maximum that, as described previously, is close to the usual sleep-onset time.[87] Thus, the paradox: the pressure to maintain wakefulness is highest just before sleep onset and the maximal drive for sleep is just before waking. The teleologic explanation is that wakefulness is maintained right up to the point of sleep onset and sleep is maintained through the night until sleep offset.

Lavie describes a "forbidden zone" for sleep.[90] Strogatz describes this as the "wake-maintenance zone".[91,92] This corresponds to the period of time just before sleep onset, when wakefulness is countered by an increasing circadian drive for sleep. There then occurs an abrupt transition from low sleep propensity during the evening period to the high-propensity night period. This time frame is called the "nocturnal sleep gate" and is found to be phase locked to the dark-phase hormone, melatonin. The "opening" of the sleep gate occurs approximately 2 hours after the time of the maximal nocturnal secretion of melatonin (**Fig. 6**).[93]

AGENTS OF ENTRAINMENT
Light

Light exposure in the early morning hours (just after the body temperature minimum) causes an advance in the sleep-wake cycle, whereas exposure to light in the early evening before the temperature minimum causes a delay in the sleep-wake cycle. Of note is that this light exposure does not have to be at the brightness level of sunlight and that even artificial incandescent light can cause phase shifts if exposure is present at critical times. It also is demonstrated that non–sleep-wake circadian rhythms are shifted by light exposure with changes in urine production, cortisol production, and melatonin secretion. All these rhythms exhibited a stable temporal relationship to temperature rhythms after light-induced phase shifts.[94,95]

Melatonin

Melatonin is synthesized from circulating tryptophan, transformed to serotonin, and then converted into melatonin in the pineal gland. There is no pineal storage of melatonin; as it is secreted, it is distributed through the circulation. Maximum plasma concentrations occur between 3:00 and 4:00 AM and during the day, levels essentially are undetectable. Even in temporal isolation, melatonin continues to express its circadian rhythm. The rhythmicity of melatonin secretion is driven by the SCN through connections to the paraventricular nuclei and then to a multisynaptic pathway that courses through the upper part of the cervical spinal cord, synapsing on preganglionic cell bodies of the superior cervical ganglia of the cervical sympathetic chains. The superior cervical ganglia then sends noradrenergic neuronal projections directly to the pineal gland.[96]

Melatonin synthesis is limited to the dark period and is inhibited by light. Exogenous melatonin exerts phase-shifting effects on the endogenous production of melatonin in humans. Melatonin administered in the morning (time of shut-down of natural melatonin production) causes phase-shift delay of the endogenous rhythm, and phase advances occur when melatonin is administered before onset of the endogenous production.

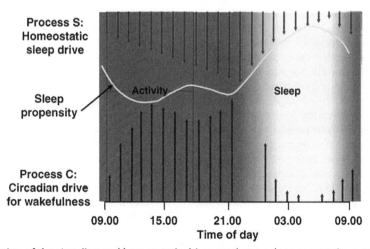

Fig. 6. The interaction of the circadian and homeostatic drives produces a sleep propensity curve that is biphasic. There is a higher sleep propensity in the midafternoon and a more robust period at night. The sleep onset occurs just after the sleep gate opens and sleep offset occurs just after the nadir of body temperature. (*Adapted from* Edgar DM, Dement W, Fuller CA. Effect of SCN lesions on sleep in squirrel monkeys: evidence for opponent processes in sleep-wake regulation. J Neurosci 1993;13:1065–79; with permission.)

It is hypothesized that the endogenous cycle of melatonin secretion is involved in the regulation of the sleep-wake cycle, not by promoting sleep actively but by inhibiting the SCN wakefulness producing mechanism.[97,98]

In this way, the evening onset of melatonin secretion, which coincides with the maximum point of the SCN-driven arousal cycle, inhibits the circadian drive for waking, enabling the sleep-onset structures to be activated, unopposed by the drive for wakefulness.

REFERENCES

1. Leadbetter R. Nyx. In: Encyclopedia mythica. Available at: Pantheon.org. 1999. Accessed April 1, 2005.
2. Poortviliet R, Huygun W. What is sleep? In: The book of the sandman and the alphabet of sleep. New York: Harry N. Abrams; 1989.
3. Rouse WHD, Smith MF. In: Lucretius: on the nature of things. Cambridge (MA): Harvard University Press; 1992. p. 34.
4. Hammond WA. Physiology of sleep: on wakefulness. Philadelphia: JB Lippincott; 1866. p. 2–38.
5. von Economo C. Sleep as a problem of localization. J Nerv Ment Dis 1930;71:249–59.
6. Aldrich MS. Neurology of sleep. In: Sleep medicine. Contemporary neurology series, vol. 53. New York: Oxford University Press; 1999. p. 27–38.
7. Berger H. Ueber das Elektroenkephalogramm des Menschen. J Psychol Neurol 1930;40:160–79.
8. Bremer F. Cerveau "isolé" et physiologie du sommeil. C R Soc Biol (Paris) 1935;118:1235–41.
9. Ramón y Cajal S. Histologie du systeme nerveux de L'homme et des vertebres maloine, vol. 2. Paris. Oxford University Press; 1911.
10. Papez JW. Reticulo-spinal tracts in the cat, Marchi method. J Comp Neurol 1926;41:365–99.
11. Morison RS, Dempsey EW. Mechanism of thalamo-cortical augmentation and repetition. Am J Physiol 1942;138:297–308.
12. de No L. The cerebral cortex: architecture, intracortical connections and motor projections. In: Fulton JF, editor. Physiology of the nervous system. London: Oxford University Press; 1938. p. 291–339.
13. Moruzzi G, Magoun HW. Communications: brain stem reticular formation and activation of the EEG. Electroencephalogr Clin Neurophysiol 1949; 1:455–73.
14. Jouvet M, Michel M. Correlations electromyographiques du sommeil chez le chat decortique et Mesencephalique chronique. C R Soc Biol (Paris) 1959; 153:422–5.
15. Jouvet M, Michel F, Courjon J. Sur un stade d'activity electrique cerebral rapide au cours du sommeil physiologique. C R Soc Biol (Paris) 1959;153: 1024–8.
16. Jouvet M, Mounier D. Effects des lesions de la formation reticulaire pontique sur le sommeil du chat. C R Soc Biol (Paris) 1960;154:2301–5.
17. Aserinsky E, Kleitman N. Regularly occurring periods of eye movements and concomitant phenomena, during sleep. Science 1953;118:273–4.
18. Aserinsky E, Kleitman N. Two types of ocular motility occurring in sleep. J Appl Physiol 1955;8:11–8.
19. Dement W, Kleitman N. Cyclic variations in EEG during sleep and their relation to eye movements, body motility and dreaming. Electroencephalogr Clin Neueophysiol 1957;9:673–90.
20. Rechtschaffen A, Kales A. A manual of standardized terminology, techniques and scoring system for sleep stages of human subjects. Los Angeles: Brain Information Service/Brain Research Institute; 1968. p. 1–12.
21. Steriade M, Gloor P, Llinás RR, et al. Basic mechanisms of cerebral rhythmic activities. Electroencephalogr Clin Neurophysiol 1990;76:481–508.
22. Colrain IM. The K-complex: a 7 decade history. Sleep 2005;28:255–73.
23. Buzsaki G, Traub RD. Physiological basis of EEG activity. In: Engel JJ, Pedley TA, editors. Epilepsy: a comprehensive textbook. New York: Raven Press; 1997. p. 819–32.
24. Steriade M, Datta S, Paré D, et al. Neuronal activities in brain-stem cholinergic nuclei related to tonic activation processes in thalamocortical systems. J Neurosci 1990;10:2541–59.
25. Pace-Schott EF, Hobson JA. The neurobiology of sleep: genetics, cellular physiology and subcortical networks. Nat Rev Neurosci 2002;3:591–605.
26. Steriade M. Arousal: revisiting the reticular activating system. Science 1996;272:225–6.
27. Armstrong DM, Saper CB, Levey AI, et al. Distribution of cholinergic neurons in rat brain: demonstrated by the immunocytochemical localization of choline acetyltransferase. J Comp Neurol 1983; 216:53–68.
28. España R, Scammell TE. Sleep neurobiology for the clinician. Sleep 2004;27:811–20.
29. Detari L, Rasmusson DD, Semba K, et al. The role of the basal forebrain neurons in tonic and phasic activation of the cerebral cortex. Prog Neurobiol 1999; 58:249.
30. Törk I. Anatomy of the serotonergic system. Ann N Y Acad Sci 1990;600:9–34.
31. Koella WP. Serotonin and sleep. Exp Med Surg 1969;27:157–68.
32. Schönrock B, Büsselberg D, Haas HL. Properties of tuberomammillary histamine neurons and their response to galanin. Agents Actions 1991;33:135–7.
33. Yang QZ, Hatton GI. Electrophysiology of excitatory and inhibitory afferents to rat histaminergic

tuberomammillary nucleus neurons from hypothalamic and forebrain sites. Brain Res 1997;773: 162–72.

34. Kilduff TS, Peyron C. The hypocretin/orexin ligand-receptor system: implications for sleep and sleep disorders. Trends Neurosci 2000;23:359–65.

35. De Lecea L, Kilduff TS, Peyron C, et al. The hypocretins: hypothalamus-specific peptides with neuroexcitatory activity. Proc Natl Acad Sci USA 1998;95: 322–7.

36. Sakurai T, Amemiya A, Ishii M, et al. Orexins and orexin receptors: a family of hypothalamic neuropeptides and G protein-coupled receptors that regulate feeding behavior. Cell 1998;92:573–85.

37. Methippara MM, Alam N, Szymusiak R, et al. Effects of lateral preoptic area application of orexin-A on sleep-wakefulness. Sleep 2000;11:3423–6.

38. España RA, Baldo BA, Kelley AE, et al. Wake-promoting and sleep-suppressing actions of hypocretin (orexin): basal forebrain sites of action. Neuroscience 2001;106:699–715.

39. Li Y, Gao XB, Sakurai T, et al. Hypocretin/orexin excites hypocretin neurons via a local glutamate neuron-a potential mechanism for orchestrating the hypothalamic arousal system. Neuron 2002;36:1169–81.

40. Torterolo P, Yamuy J, Sampogna S, et al. Hypothalamic neurons that contain hypocretin (orexin) express c-fos during active wakefulness and carbachol-induced active sleep. Available at: www. sro.org. Accessed March 15, 2005. Sleep Res Online 2001;4:25–32.

41. Morrison JH, Foote SL. Noradrenergic and serotoninergic innervation of cortical, thalamic and tectal visual structures in Old and New World monkeys. J Comp Neurol 1986;243:117–38.

42. Tasaka K, Chung YH, Sawada K. Excitatory effect of histamine on the arousal system and its inhibition by H1 blockers. Brain Res Bull 1989;22:271–5.

43. Mignot E, Taheri S, Nishino S. Sleeping with the hypothalamus: emerging therapeutic targets for sleep disorders. Nat Neurosci 2002;5:1071–5.

44. Hillarp NA, Fuxe K, Dahlström A. Demonstration and mapping of central neurons containing dopamine, noradrenalin, and 5-hydroxytryptamine and their reactions to psychopharmaca. Pharmacol Rev 1966;18:727–39.

45. Dzoljic MR, Ukponmwan OE, Saxena PR. 5–HT1-like receptor agonists enhance wakefulness. Neuropharmacology 1992;31:623–33.

46. Nishino S, Mao J, Sampathkumaran R, et al. Increased dopaminergic transmission mediates the wake-promoting effects of CNS stimulants. Sleep Res Online 1998;1:49–61. Available at: www.sro. org. Accessed March 15, 2005.

47. Wisor JP, Nishino S, Sora I, et al. Dopaminergic role in stimulant-induced wakefulness. J Neurosci 2001; 21:1787–94.

48. Isaac SO, Berridge CW. Wake-promoting actions of dopamine D1 and D2 receptor stimulation. J Phamacol Exp Ther 2003;307:386–94.

49. Rye DB. The two faces of Eve: dopamine's modulation of wakefulness and sleep. Neurology 2004;63. 8 (Suppl 3):S2-7.

50. Lin L, Faraco J, Li R, et al. The sleep disorder canine narcolepsy is caused by a mutation in the hypocretin (orexin) receptor 2 gene. Cell 1999;98:365–76.

51. Chemelli RM, Willie JT, Sinton CM, et al. Narcolepsy in orexin knockout mice: molecular genetics of sleep regulation. Cell 1999;98:437–51.

52. Siegel JM, Moore R, Thannickal T, et al. A brief history of hypocretin/orexin and narcolepsy. Neuropyshophamacology 2001;25(S5):S14–20.

53. Thannickal TC, Moore RY, Nienhuis R, et al. Reduced number of hypocretin neurons in human narcolepsy. Neuron 2000;27:469–74.

54. Kisanuki YY, Chemelli RM, Sinton CM, et al. The role of orexin receptor type-1 (OX1R) in the regulation of sleep. Sleep 2000;A91.

55. Sherin JE, Shiromani PJ, McCarley RW, et al. Activation of ventrolateral preoptic neurons during sleep. Science 1996;271:216–9.

56. Porkka-Heiskanen T, Strecker RE, Thakkar M, et al. Adenosine: a mediator of the sleep-inducing effects of prolonged wakefulness. Science 1997;276:1265–8.

57. Tanase D, Martin WA, Baghdoyan HA, et al. G protein activation in rat ponto-mesencephalic nuclei is enhanced by combined treatment with a mu opioid and an adenosine A1 receptor agonist. Sleep 2001;24:52–61.

58. Chamberlin NL, Arrigoni E, Chou TC, et al. Effects of adenosine on GABAergic synaptic inputs to identified ventrolateral preoptic neurons. Neuroscience 2003;119:913–8.

59. Ueno R, Ishikawa Y, Nakayama T, et al. Prostaglandin D2 induces sleep when microinjected into the preoptic area of conscious rats. Biochem Biophys Res Commun 1982;109:576–82.

60. Saper CB, Chou TC, Scammell TE. The sleep switch: hypothalamic control of sleep and wakefulness. Trends Neurosci 2001;24:726–31.

61. EL Mansari M, Saaki K, Jouvet M. Unitary characteristics of presumptive cholinergic tegmental neurons during the sleep-waking cycle in freely moving cats. Exp Brain Res 1989;76:519–29.

62. Boissard R, Gervasoni D, Schmidt MH, et al. The rat ponto-medullary network responsible for paradoxical sleep onset and maintenance: a combined microinjection and functional neuroanatomy study. Eur J Neurosci 2002;16:1959–73.

63. Morales FR, Engelhardt JK, Soja PJ, et al. Motoneuroneuron properties during motor inhibition produced by microinjection of carbachol into the pontine reticular formation of the decerebrate cat. J Neurophysiol 1987;57:1118–29.

64. Sinton CM, McCarley RW. Neurophysiological mechanisms of sleep and wakefulness: a question of balance. SeminNeurol 2004;24:211–23.

65. Saper CB. Neurobiology of sleep. In: Education program syllabus. American Academy of Neurology, 57th meeting. 2005. p. 3AC.001-1-3.

66. Curtis DR, Hosli L, Johnston GA, et al. The hyperpolarization of spinal motorneurons by glycine and related amino acids. Exp Brain Res 1968;5:235–58.

67. Johnson RF, Moore RY, Morin LP. Loss of entrainment and anatomical plasticity after lesions of the hamster retinohypothalamic tract. Brain Res 1988; 460:297–313.

68. Berson DM, Dunn FA, Tako M. Phototransduction by retinal ganglion cells that act the circadian clock. Science 2002;295:1070–3.

69. Morin LP. Serotonin and the regulation of mammalian circadian rhythmicity. Ann Med 1999;31:12–33.

70. Bina KG, Rusak B, Semba K. Localization of cholinergic neurons in the forebrain and brainstem that project to the suprachiasmatic nucleus of the hypothalamus in rat. J Comp Neurol 1993;335:295–307.

71. Moore RY, Card JP. Intergeniculate leaflet: an anatomically and functionally distinct subdivision of the lateral genicuilate complex. J Comp Neurol 1994;344:403–30.

72. Morin LP. The circadian visual system. Brain Res Rev 1994;67:102–27.

73. Harrington ME, Mistlberger RE. Anatomy and physiology of the mammalian circadian system. In: Fryger MH, Roth T, Dement WC, editors. Principles and practice of sleep medicine. 2nd edition. Philadelphia: WB Saunders; 2000. p. 334–45.

74. Biello SM, Janik D, Mrfosovsky N. Neuropeptide Y and behaviorally induced phase shifts. Neuroscience 1994;62:273–9.

75. Watts AG, Swanson LW. Efferent projections of the suprachiasmatic nucleus, II: studies using retrograde transport of fluorescent dyes and simultaneous peptide immunochemistry in the rat. J Comp Neurol 1987;258:230–52.

76. Konopka RJ, Benzer S. Clock mutants of Drosophila melanogaster. Proc Natl Acad Sci USA 1971;68: 2112–6.

77. Albrecht U. Functional genomics of sleep and circadian rhythm. Invited review: regulation of mammalian circadian clock genes. J Appl Physiol 2002;92:1348–55.

78. Daan S, Beersma DG, Borbely AA. Timing of human sleep recovery process gated by a circadian pacemaker. Am J Physiology 1984;246:161–83.

79. Borbély AA, Tobler I. Endogenous sleep-promoting substances and sleep regulation. Physiol Rev 1989;69:605–58.

80. Legendre R, Pieron H. Le probleme des facteurs du sommeil. Resultats d'injections vasculaires et intracerebrales de liquids insomniques. C R Soc Biol (Paris) 1910;68:1077–9.

81. Späth-Schwalbe E, Lange T, Perras B, et al. Interferon-α acutely impairs sleep in healthy humans. Cytokine 2000;12:518–21.

82. Blake MJF. Time of day effects on performance in a range of tasks. Psychonom Sci 1967;9:349–50.

83. Webb WB, Agnew HW, Williams RL. Effects on sleep of a sleep period time displacement. Aerosp Med 1971;42:152–5.

84. Aschoff J, Wever R. Spotanperiodik des menschen bei ausschluss aller zeitgeber. Naturwissenschaften 1962;49:337–42.

85. Zulley J. Distribution of REM sleep in entrained 24 hour and free-running sleep-wake cycles. Sleep 1980;2:377–89.

86. Zulley J, Wever R, Aschoff J. The dependence of onset and duration of sleep on the circadian rhythm of rectal temperature. Pflugers Arch 1981; 391:314–8.

87. Czeisler CA, Zimmerman JC, Ronda JM, et al. Timing of REM sleep is coupled to the circadian rhythm of body temperature in man. Sleep 1980;2: 329–46.

88. Zulley J, Campbell SS. Napping behavior during spontaneous internal desynchronization: sleep remains in synchrony with body temperature. Human Neurobiology 1985;4:123–6.

89. Lavie P. Sleep-wake as a biological rhythm. Annu Rev Psychol 2001;52:277–303.

90. Lavie P. Ultrashort sleep-waking schedule: III. 'Gates' and 'forbidden zones' for sleep. Electroencephal Clin Neurophysiol 1986;63:414–25.

91. Strogatz SH. The mathematical structure of the human sleep wake cycle. New York: Springer-Verlag; 1986.

92. Liu X, Uchiyama M, Shibui K, et al. Diurnal preference, sleep habits, circadian sleep propensity and melatonin rhytm in healthy human subjects. Neurosci Lett 2000;280:199–202.

93. Fröberg J. Twenty-four hour patterns in human performance, subjective and physiological variables and differences between morning and evening types. Biol Psychol 1977;5:119–34.

94. Czeisler CA, Allan JS, Strogatz SH, et al. Bright light resets the human circadian pacemaker independent of the timing of the sleep-wake cycle. Science 1986; 233:667–71.

95. Czeisler CA, Kronauer RE, Allan JS, et al. Bright light induction of strong (type 0) resetting of the human circadian pacemaker. Science 1989;244:1328–33.

96. Arendt J. Melatonin and the mammalian pineal gland. London: Chapman-Hall; 1995.

97. Lewy AJ, Ahmed S, Jackson JM, Sack RL. Melatonin shifts human circadian rhythms according to a phase-response curve. Chronobiol Int 1992;9: 380–92.

98. Lavie P. Melatonin: role in gating nocturnal rise in sleep propensity. J Biol Rhythms 1997;12:657–65.

Learning, Memory, and Sleep in Humans

Jessica D. Payne, PhD

KEYWORDS

- Slow wave sleep • Memory • Hippocampus
- Rapid eye movement sleep

About one-third of a person's life is spent sleeping, yet in spite of the advances in understanding the processes that generate and maintain sleep, the functional significance of sleep remains a mystery. Numerous theories regarding the role of sleep have been proposed, including homeostatic restoration, thermoregulation, tissue repair, and immune control. A theory that has received enormous support in the last decade concerns sleep's role in processing and storing memories. This article reviews some of the evidence suggesting that sleep is critical for long-lasting memories. This body of evidence has grown impressively large and covers a range of studies at the molecular, cellular, physiologic, and behavioral levels of analysis.

DEFINING SLEEP AND MEMORY
Stages of Sleep

There are 2 main types of sleep. The first, rapid eye movement (REM) sleep, occurs in roughly 90-minute cycles throughout the night and alternates with 4 additional stages (stages 1–4) known collectively as non-REM (NREM) sleep, which comprises the second type of sleep.[1] Slow wave sleep (SWS) is the deepest of the NREM sleep phases and is characterized by high-amplitude, low-frequency oscillations seen in the electroencephalogram (EEG). REM sleep, on the other hand, is a lighter stage of sleep characterized by rapid eye movements (REMs), decreased muscle tone, and low-amplitude fast EEG oscillations. More than 80% of SWS is concentrated in the first half of the typical 8-hour night, whereas the second half of the night contains roughly twice as much REM sleep than the first half (**Fig. 1**).

This domination of early sleep by SWS and of late sleep by REM sleep not only has important functional consequences but also makes it difficult to know which distinction is critical for memory processing: NREM versus REM sleep or early versus late sleep.

Neurotransmitters, particularly the monoamines serotonin (5-HT) and norepinephrine (NE), and acetylcholine (ACh), play a critical role in switching the brain from one sleep stage to another. REM sleep occurs when activity in the aminergic system has decreased enough to allow the reticular system to escape its inhibitory influence.[1] The release from aminergic inhibition stimulates cholinergic reticular neurons in the brainstem and switches the sleeping brain into the highly active REM state, in which ACh levels are as high as in the waking state. Overall, REM sleep is also associated with higher levels of cortisol than NREM sleep. 5-HT and NE, on the other hand, are virtually absent during REM sleep. SWS, conversely, is associated with an absence of ACh and low levels of cortisol but detectable levels of 5-HT and NE.[2,3]

Stages of Memory Formation, and Different Memory Types

Memory consolidation is the process by which newly acquired information, initially fragile, is integrated and stabilized into long-term memory.[4] Evidence overwhelmingly suggests that sleep plays a role in the consolidation of a range of memory tasks, with the different stages of sleep selectively benefiting the consolidation of different types of memory.[2,5–10]

Like sleep, memory is also divided into several key stages and types.[11] First, there are various types of memories that can be recalled explicitly, including episodic memories, or memories of the

Department of Psychology, University of Notre Dame, Haggar Hall, Room 122-B, Notre Dame, Indiana 46556, USA
E-mail address: Jessica.payne.70@nd.edu

Sleep Med Clin 6 (2011) 15–30
doi:10.1016/j.jsmc.2010.12.005
1556-407X/11/$ – see front matter © 2011 Elsevier Inc. All rights reserved.

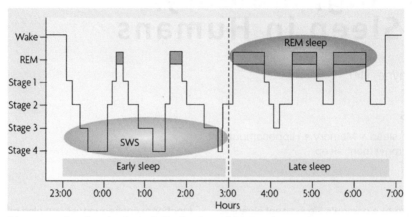

Fig. 1. A sleep histogram showing the typical distribution of SWS and REM sleep.

events in our lives. Retrieving an episodic memory from one's past requires access to defining contextual features of the event, such as specific details about the place and time of its occurrence. Because of this emphasis on spatial context, episodic memories and spatial memories are closely connected. Second, there are semantic memories, which are concerned with the knowledge one acquires during events but is itself separated from the specific event in question. Thus, our knowledge about the meaning of words and facts about the world, even though acquired in the context of some specific experience, appears to be stored in a context-independent format (eg, not bound to the originating context). Third, there are "how to" memories for the various skills, procedures, and habits that we acquire through experience. Because these memories are not so easily made explicit and are usually only evident in behavior, they are referred to as procedural or implicit memories. Finally, there are emotional memories for the positive and negative experiences in our lives. This class of memories is especially concerned with learning about fearful and negative stimuli, although evidence suggests it plays a role in learning about pleasant information as well.[12]

Evidence suggests that each of these memory types is subserved by distinct neural systems.[11–13] Whereas episodic and spatial memories are governed by the hippocampus and surrounding medial temporal areas, procedural or implicit memories are thought to be independent of the hippocampus and anatomically related regions, relying instead on various neocortical and subcortical structures. The emotional memory system is centered in the amygdala, a limbic structure that is richly connected to the hippocampus.[14] Importantly, evidence suggests that information dependent on each of these systems is processed

differently during sleep. Although somewhat oversimplified,[15] there is a general consensus that NREM sleep, especially SWS, is important for the consolidation of explicit episodic and spatial memories, both of which rely on the hippocampus for their consolidation,[16] whereas REM sleep selectively benefits procedural and emotional memories.[17,18]

In addition to these distinct types, memory consolidation also consists of different stages. Although our experience of memory occurs at the moment of retrieval when information about the initial experience returns to conscious awareness, successful retrieval is contingent on the successful completion of at least 2 earlier stages of memory formation. First, the experience or information must be properly encoded. Encoding involves transforming new information into a representation capable of being stored in memory, just as the key presses that are made on a keyboard must be converted to a format that can be stored in a computer. Second, the information must be consolidated or durably stored in a manner that can withstand the passage of time. Only if these processes occur successfully will it be possible for information from the initial event to be retrieved later in time. Although this article mostly focuses on memory consolidation, it also briefly reviews new evidence that sleep is essential for effective memory encoding.

SLEEP BENEFITS IMPLICIT AND PROCEDURAL MEMORIES

Sleep seems to benefit the consolidation of both implicit and explicit forms of memory. Converging data suggest that most procedural skills and abilities (eg, performing a surgery, riding a bike) are acquired slowly and are not attained solely during the learning episode. While some learning certainly develops quickly, performance on various procedural tasks improves further and without additional practice simply through the passage of time, particularly if these periods contain sleep. These slow off-line improvements occur as newly acquired information, initially fragile, is integrated and stabilized into long-term memory.

Early work investigating the effect of sleep on implicit learning used a visual texture discrimination task (VDT) originally developed by Karni and Sagi.[19] The task requires participants to determine the orientation (vertical or horizontal) of an array of diagonal bars that is embedded in one visual quadrant against a background of exclusively horizontal bars (**Fig. 2**). At the center of the screen is the fixation target, which is either the letter *T* or the letter *L*. This target screen is succeeded first by a blank screen for a variable interstimulus interval (ISI) and then by a mask (a screen covered with randomly oriented *V*'s with a superimposed *T* and *L* in the center). Subjects must determine the orientation of the array, and the performance is estimated by the ISI corresponding to 80% correct responses.[19,20]

Amnesic patients with damage to the hippocampal complex, who cannot acquire knowledge explicitly, show normal performance improvements on the VDT.[21] In neurologically normal subjects, improvement on the VDT develops slowly after training,[19,22] with no improvement when retesting occurs on the same day as training (**Fig. 3A**). Instead, improvement is only observed after a night of sleep (see **Fig. 3A**). This observation was true even for a group of subjects who were retested only 9 hours after training. Importantly, there was not even a trend to greater improvement when the training-retest interval was increased from 9.0 to 22.5 hours, suggesting that additional wake time after the night of sleep provided no additional benefit. Whereas further wake time provided no benefit, additional nights of sleep did produce incremental improvement. When subjects were retested 2 to 7 days after training rather than after a single night of sleep

a 50% greater improvement was observed (see **Fig. 3B**). Critically, another group of subjects was sleep deprived on the first night after training. These subjects were allowed 2 full nights of recovery sleep before being retested 3 days later. The subjects failed to show any residual learning, suggesting that performance enhancements depend on a normal first night of sleep (see **Fig. 3B**). Time alone is clearly not enough to produce long-term benefits from VDT training. It seems that sleep is also required.[22]

Initially, improvement on this task seemed to depend solely on REM sleep, because subjects who underwent selective deprivation of REM sleep showed no improvement on the task.[20] Later studies, however, showed that optimal performance on this task requires both SWS and REM sleep.[23]

When subjects were trained and their subsequent sleep monitored in the sleep laboratory, the amount of improvement was proportional to the amount of SWS during the first quarter of the night (**Fig. 4A**), as well as to the amount of REM sleep in the last quarter (see **Fig. 4B**). Indeed, the product of these 2 sleep parameters explained more than 80% of the intersubject variance (see **Fig. 4D**). No significant correlations were found for sleep stage during other parts of the night (see **Fig. 4C**) or for the amount of stage 2 sleep at any time during the night.

Gais and colleagues[24] came to a similar conclusion by examining improvement after 3 hours of sleep either early or late in the night. They found that 3 hours of early night sleep, which was rich in SWS, produced an 8-millisecond improvement, but after a full night of sleep, which added REM-rich sleep late in the night, a 26-millisecond improvement was observed, 3 times that seen with early sleep alone. However, 3 hours of REM-rich, late night sleep actually produced deterioration in performance.[24] These results are further corroborated by daytime nap studies. Afternoon naps as short as 60 to 90 minutes also lead to

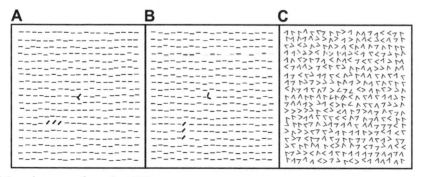

Fig. 2. (*A–C*) Sample screens from the VDT.

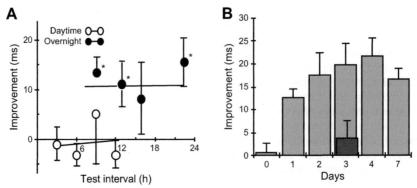

Fig. 3. Sleep-dependent improvement on the VDT. All subjects were trained and then retested only once. Each point in (A) and each green bar in (B) represents a separate group of subjects. Error bars in (A) and (B) are SEM. (A) There was no improvement when retesting occurred on the same day as training (*open circles*), but there was improvement after a night of sleep (*closed circles*). Asterisks indicate significant effects. (B) (*Green bars*) Improvement in performance of subjects when retested 2 to 7 days of training. (*Red bar*) No improvement in performance of subjects who were sleep deprived on the first night of training. ms, milliseconds. (*From* Stickgold R, James L, Hobson JA. Visual discrimination learning requires post-training sleep. Nat Neurosci 2000;2 (12):1237–8; with permission; and Stickgold R, Whidbee D, Schirmer B, et al. Visual discrimination task improvement: a multi-step process occurring during sleep. J Cognit Neurosci 2000;12:246–54; with permission.)

performance benefits on the VDT, especially when they contain REM and NREM sleep.[25,26]

At this point, sleep's role in visual discrimination learning (as measured by VDT performance) is clear. But the VDT represents a very specific type of sensory memory that may or may not share its sleep dependency with other procedural tasks. This specificity raises the question of whether the sleep effects observed with the VDT generalize to other forms of procedural memory. Studies of

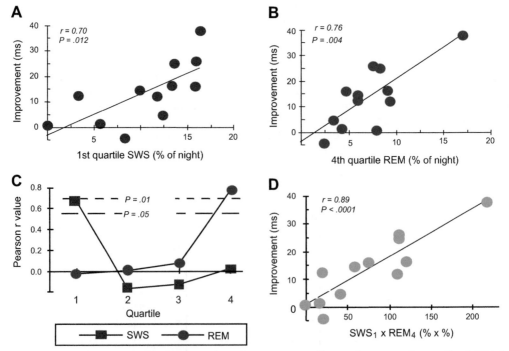

Fig. 4. (*A–D*) REM sleep and SWS dependence of VDT learning. ms, milliseconds; REM$_4$, 4th quartile of REM sleep; SWS$_1$, 1st quartile of SWS. (*From* Stickgold R, Whidbee D, Schirmer B, et al. Visual discrimination task improvement: a multi-step process occurring during sleep. J Cognit Neurosci 2000;12:246–54; with permission.)

sleep-dependent motor skill learning strongly suggest that they do.

As an example, Walker and colleagues[27] have demonstrated sleep-dependent improvements on a finger tapping task. The task requires subjects to repeatedly type the numeric sequence 4-1-3-2-4 as quickly and accurately as possible with the non-dominant hand. Training consisted of twelve 30-second trials separated by 30-second rest periods. All subjects show considerable improvement during the 12 trials of the training session (a fast learning component), but 12 hours later, the subjects performed differently depending on whether the 12-hour interval was spent sleeping or awake. When trained in the morning and retested 12 hours later, only an additional nonsignificant 4% improvement was seen in performance, but when tested again the next morning, a large and robust (14%) improvement was seen (**Fig. 5A**). The failure to improve during the daytime could not be caused by interference from related motor activity because subjects who were required to wear mittens and refrain from fine motor activities during this time showed a similar pattern of wake/sleep improvement (see **Fig. 5B**).

In contrast, when subjects were trained in the evening, improvement was observed the following morning (after sleep) but not across an additional 12 hours of wake (see **Fig. 5C**). Thus, improved performance resulted specifically from a night of sleep as opposed to the simple passage of time. Curiously, unlike the findings for the VDT, overnight improvement on this task correlated with the amount of stage 2 NREM sleep during the night, especially during the last quarter of the night.

These findings are in agreement with those of Fogel and colleagues,[28] Smith and MacNeill,[29] and Tweed and colleagues,[30] who have also shown that stage 2 sleep and possibly the sleep spindles that reach peak density during late night stage 2 sleep are critical for simple motor memory consolidation. This role of sleep spindles seems plausible because they have been proposed to trigger intracellular mechanisms that are required for synaptic plasticity.[31]

This motor sequence task has been examined to determine where precisely in the motor program this sleep-dependent improvement occurs.[32] In the sequence mentioned earlier (4-1-3-2-4), there are 4 unique key-press transitions: 4 to 1, 1 to 3, 3 to 2, and 2 to 4. When the speed between transitions was analyzed for individual subjects before sleep, "sticking points" emerged. Whereas some transitions were easy (ie, fast), others were problematic (ie, slow), as if the sequence was being parsed or chunked into smaller bits during presleep learning.[21] After a night of sleep, these problematic points were preferentially improved, whereas transitions that had already been mastered before sleep did not change. Subjects who were trained and retested after a daytime wake interval showed no such improvements.

These findings suggest that the sleep-dependent consolidation process involves the

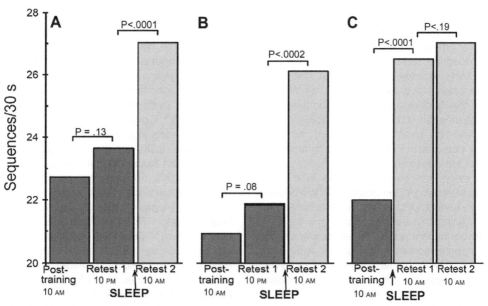

Fig. 5. (*A–C*) Sleep-dependent motor learning. Improvement in speed was seen in all 3 groups over a night of sleep but not over 12 hours of daytime wake. (*From* Walker M, Brakefield T, Morgan A, et al. Practice with sleep makes perfect: sleep dependent motor skill learning. Neuron 2002;35:205–11; with permission.)

unification of smaller motor memory units into a single motor memory representation, thereby improving problem points in the sequence. Importantly, this finding suggests that the role of sleep is subtle and complex and that sleep does more than simply strengthen memories; sleep may encourage the restructuring and reorganization of memories, an important and often-overlooked aspect of memory consolidation. The author returns to this idea later in the article.

Moving to another type of motor memory, motor adaptation, Maquet and colleagues[33] showed that sleep benefits performance on a motor pursuit task. Participants were trained to use a joystick to keep the cursor on a target when the target trajectory was predictable only on the horizontal axis, which meant that optimal performance could only be achieved by developing an implicit model of the motion characteristics of the learned trajectory. Half of the subjects were sleep deprived on the first posttraining night, whereas the other half were allowed to sleep normally. Three days later, after 2 full nights of recovery sleep, performance was superior in the sleep group compared with the sleep-deprived group, and functional magnetic resonance imaging (fMRI) revealed that that the superior temporal sulcus (STS) was differentially more active for the learned trajectory in subjects who slept than in the sleep-deprived subjects. Moreover, increased functional connectivity was observed between the STS and the cerebellum and between the supplementary and frontal eye fields, suggestive of sleep-related plastic changes during motor skill consolidation in areas involved in smooth pursuit and eye movements.

Admittedly, visual discrimination, finger tapping, and motor adaptation are all relatively basic low-level procedural tasks that may become automated fairly quickly. What about the more complex implicit and procedural tasks? Work on animals clearly demonstrates that complex tasks (eg, instrumental conditioning, avoidance, or maze learning) benefit from sleep, with rats showing increases in REM sleep that continue until the tasks are mastered.[34–36]

REM sleep has been implicated in complex procedural learning in humans as well. In a positron emission tomographic study of visuomotor skill memory using the serial reaction time task,[37] 6 spatially permanent position markers were shown on a computer screen and subjects watched for stimuli to appear below these markers. When a stimulus appeared in a particular position, subjects reacted as quickly as possible by pressing a corresponding key on the keyboard. Because the stimuli were generated in an order defined by a probabilistic finite-state grammar,

improvement on the task (compared with randomly generated sequences) reflects implicitly acquired knowledge of this grammar.[37]

Neuroimaging was performed on 3 groups of subjects. One group was scanned while they were awake, both at rest and during performance of the task, providing information about which brain regions are typically activated by the task. A second group of subjects was trained on the task during the afternoon and then scanned the night after training, both while awake and during various sleep stages. Thus, group 2 was included to determine if similar brain regions were reactivated during sleep. A postsleep session was also conducted to verify that learning had indeed occurred. Finally, a third group, never trained on the task, was scanned while sleeping to ensure that the pattern of activation present in natural sleep was different from the pattern of activation present after training.

Results showed that during REM sleep, as compared with resting wakefulness, several brain areas used during task performance were more active in trained than in nontrained subjects. These areas included occipital, parietal, anterior cingulate, motor, and premotor cortices and the cerebellum, all activations that are consistent with the component processes involved in the visual and motor functioning involved in this task. Behavioral data confirmed that trained subjects improved significantly more across the night.

Peigneux and colleagues,[38] using the same task, showed that the level of acquisition of probabilistic rules attained before sleep was correlated with the increase in activation of task-related cortical areas during posttraining REM sleep. This observation suggests that cerebral reactivation is modulated by the strength of the memory traces developed during the learning episode, and as such, these data provide the first experimental evidence linking behavioral performance to reactivation during REM sleep.[38] Together with animal studies,[39,40] these findings suggest that it is not simply experiencing the task, but the process of memory consolidation associated with successful learning of the task that modifies sleep physiology.

These results support the idea that implicit/procedural memory traces in humans can be reactivated during REM sleep, and that this reactivation is linked to improved consolidation. Indeed, looking a bit more closely at the literature, human REM sleep has also been linked to memory for complex logic games, to foreign language acquisition, and to intensive studying.[41] It is interesting that these more-complex conceptual-procedural tasks often show REM sleep relationships, whereas more basic procedural tasks benefit mainly from NREM sleep. The above-mentioned findings provide encouraging evidence that sleep-based processes can aid in procedural memory consolidation, not only for basic forms of sensory and motor memory in humans but also for complex procedural and conceptual knowledge. Moreover, these findings indicate that the consolidation of familiar skills, or those that are similar to other well-learned skills, may be reliant on NREM sleep stages (particularly stage 2 NREM sleep), whereas REM sleep may be required for the integration of new concepts or skills with preexisting information stored in memory.[42] This is an important concept that warrants future investigation.

Clearly, sleep is crucial to the consolidation of procedural memory. Although both the stabilization of explicitly learned motor skills and off-line improvements in pure implicit tasks may evolve over time spent awake,[43,44] the posttraining enhancement of motor skills seems to be exclusively dependent on sleep.[27] Participants with insomnia show impaired sleep-related procedural memory consolidation compared with participants with undisturbed sleep,[45] and schizophrenia, which is associated with changes in sleep, particularly in stage 2 NREM sleep spindles,[46,47] is also associated with procedural memory deficits.[48] More recently, Dresler and colleagues[49] demonstrated that off-line procedural memory consolidation is also disturbed in depression, another condition associated with changes in sleep architecture.

SLEEP BENEFITS EXPLICIT MEMORIES

This section describes the relationship between sleep and the consolidation of explicit memories.

There is a general consensus that NREM sleep, especially SWS, is important for the consolidation of hippocampus-dependent episodic and spatial memories.[16] In a landmark study, Plihal and Born[50] assessed the recall of word pairs (an episodic memory task) and improvement in mirror tracing (a procedural memory task) after retention intervals of early sleep (the first 3–4 hours of the sleep cycle), which, as noted in the previous sections, is dominated by SWS, and late sleep (the last 3–4 hours of the sleep cycle), which is dominated by REM sleep. Recall of word pairs improved more significantly after a 3-hour sleep period rich in SWS than after a 3-hour sleep period rich in REM sleep or a 3-hour period of wakefulness. Mirror tracing, on the other hand, improved significantly more after a 3-hour sleep period rich in REM sleep than after 3 hours spent either in SWS or awake.

Similarly, using a nap paradigm, Tucker and colleagues[51] found that naps containing only NREM sleep enhanced memory for word pairs but did not benefit mirror tracing. After an afternoon training session, performance on these tasks was assessed after a 6-hour delay, either with or without an intervening nap. The subjects who were allowed a nap not only recalled more word pairs than the subjects who remained awake (**Fig. 6**) but also showed a weak correlation between improved recall and the amount of SWS in the nap.

These results are consistent with neurophysiological evidence derived from electrophysiological studies in rodents, which demonstrate that patterns of hippocampal place cell activity first seen during waking exploration are later reexpressed during postlearning SWS.[52–54] Similarly,

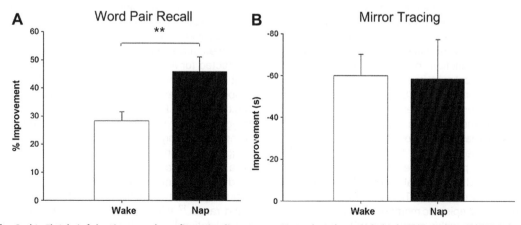

Fig. 6. (*A, B*) A brief daytime nap benefits episodic memory. Note that the nap (which did not contain REM sleep) benefited episodic, but not procedural memory. Asterisks indicate significant differences between groups. (*From* Tucker MA, Hirota Y, Wamsley EJ, et al. A daytime nap containing solely non-REM sleep enhances declarative but not procedural memory. Neurobiol Learn Mem 2006;86(2):241–7; with permission.)

several neuroimaging studies in humans have suggested an important role for SWS in hippocampus-dependent memory consolidation. The first of these studies investigated performance on a hippocampally-dependent virtual maze task.[55] Daytime learning of the task was associated with hippocampal activity. During posttraining sleep, there was a reemergence of hippocampal activation, and this activation occurred specifically during SWS. The most compelling finding, however, is that the increase in hippocampal activation seen during posttraining SWS was proportional to the amount of improvement seen the next day. This finding suggests that the reexpression of hippocampal activation during SWS reflects the off-line reprocessing of spatial episodic memory traces, which in turn leads to the plastic changes underlying the improvement in memory performance seen the next day. Similarly, Rasch and colleagues[56] exposed human subjects to an odor while they were learning object-location pairings in a task similar to the memory game "concentration;" subjects who were reexposed to the odor during SWS (but not REM sleep) showed enhanced hippocampal activity and enhanced memory for the memory pairings.

Another study[57] investigated the time course of episodic memory consolidation across 90 days. Subjects studied 360 photographs of landscapes and were then tested on subsets of the photographs either after a nap the same day or after 2, 30, or 90 days. Before each test, subjects studied 80 new pictures and then were tested on 80 of the original pictures and the 80 new ones as well as 80 pictures that they had never seen before. All memory retrieval sessions occurred during fMRI scanning. After the initial 90-minute nap, stage 2 sleep was positively correlated with successful recall of both remote and recent items, indicating a nonspecific benefit of stage 2 NREM sleep on episodic memory. This is an intriguing finding, given that stage 2 is when sleep spindles are most prominent (see section on neurophysiological and neurochemical evidence for sleep's role in memory consolidation later). SWS, on the other hand, was correlated only with memory for remote (but not recent) items. Because performance on remote items increased with longer SWS duration, but performance for recent items did not, the effect on memory performance for remote items cannot be explained by a general effect of SWS on memory retrieval processes. These findings strongly suggest that episodic memories can undergo initial consolidation within a rather short time frame and that this consolidation is promoted by SWS.

These observations suggest that learning triggers the reactivation of episodic memory traces during NREM SWS, a process that in turn enhances behavioral performance.

SLEEP BENEFITS EMOTIONAL MEMORY CONSOLIDATION

Sleep also contributes to the consolidation of emotional episodic memories. As noted in the previous section, sleep clearly benefits memory for neutral episodic memory materials across both verbal and spatial modalities.[5,16] However, when emotional (especially emotionally negative) episodic items are intermixed with neutral items in a study, sleep disproportionately benefits the consolidation of emotional memories relative to neutral memories. For example, Hu and colleagues[58] examined the effect of a full night's sleep on both axes of emotional affect, valence (positive/negative) and arousal (high/low), across both "remember" and "know" judgments of memory for pictures. Results showed that a night of sleep improved memory accuracy for emotionally arousing pictures relative to an equivalent period of daytime wakefulness, but only for know judgments. No differences were observed for remember judgments. Moreover, memory bias changed across a night of sleep relative to wake, such that subjects became more conservative when making remember judgments, especially for emotionally arousing pictures. No bias differences were observed for know judgments between sleep and wake.

REM sleep may be particularly important for the consolidation of emotional memories, which rely critically on the amygdala for their consolidation.[7,59] Wagner and colleagues[59] found that 3 hours of late night REM-rich sleep (but not 3 hours of early night slow wave–rich sleep or 3 hours of wakefulness) facilitated memory for negative arousing narratives, an effect that could still be observed years later when the subjects were recontacted for a follow-up memory test.[60] Consistent with these findings, the amygdala and hippocampus are among the most active brain regions during REM sleep, with some evidence suggesting that they are more active during REM sleep than during wakefulness.[61] This observation suggests that emotional memory processing may be a primary goal of REM sleep. Moreover, several studies have correlated features of REM sleep, including oscillatory activity in the theta frequency band range,[17] with enhanced emotional memory consolidation.[10,62] These findings strongly suggest a role for sleep, especially REM sleep, in the processing of memory for emotional experiences.

SLEEP TRANSFORMS MEMORIES IN USEFUL WAYS

The findings reviewed in the previous sections provide compelling evidence that sleep plays an important role in solidifying experience into long-term memory in a veridical manner, more or less true to its form at initial encoding.[63] However, it has long been known that memories change with the passage of time,[64] suggesting that the process of consolidation does not always yield exact representations of past experiences. On the face of it, this process may seem strikingly maladaptive, yet such flexibility in memory representation allows the emergence of key cognitive abilities, such as generalization and inference,[65] future thought,[66] and selective preservation of useful information extracted from a barrage of incoming stimulations and experiences.[67,68] Consistent with these ideas, growing evidence suggests that sleep does more than simply consolidating memories in a veridical form; it also transforms them in ways rendering the memories less accurate in some respects but more useful and adaptive in the long run. Sleep leads to flexible restructuring of memory traces so that insights can be made,[69] inferences can be drawn,[64] and both integration and abstraction can occur.[68] In each of these cases, sleep confers a flexibility to memory that may at times be more advantageous than a literal representation of experience.

As a specific example of such qualitative changes in memory representation, recent studies demonstrate that sleep transforms the emotional memory trace. Payne and colleagues[7,67] examined how the different components of complex negative arousing memories change across periods of sleep versus wakefulness. Emotional scenes could be stored as intact units, suffering some forgetting over time but retaining the same relative vividness for all components. Alternatively, the components of an experience could undergo differential memory processing, perhaps with a selective emphasis on what is most salient and worthy of remembering.

Participants viewed scenes depicting negative or neutral objects embedded on neutral backgrounds at 9 AM or 9 PM. Twelve hours later, after a day spent awake or a night including at least 6 hours of sleep, they were tested on their memory for objects and backgrounds separately to examine how these individual components of emotional memories change across periods of sleep and wake (see **Fig. 7** for example stimuli).

Daytime wakefulness led to forgetting of negative arousing scenes in their entirety, with both objects and backgrounds being forgotten at similar rates. Sleep, however, led to a selective preservation of negative objects but not their accompanying backgrounds, suggesting that the 2 components undergo differential processing during sleep. This finding suggests that rather than preserving intact representations of scenes the sleeping brain effectively unbinds scenes to consolidate only their most emotionally salient, and perhaps adaptive, elements (see[68,69] for additional examples of potential unbinding during sleep).

Paralleling these behavioral findings, a recent fMRI study provided evidence that a single night of sleep is sufficient to provoke changes in the emotional memory circuitry, leading to increased

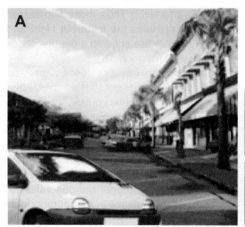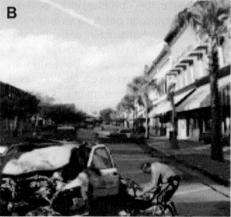

Fig. 7. Example stimuli for emotional trade-off task, where a neutral (intact car, *A*) or negative (crashed car, *B*) object is embedded on a neutral background scene (street). (*From* Payne JD, Kensinger EA. Sleep's role in the consolidation of emotional episodic memories. Curr Dir Psychol Sci 2010;19(5):290–5; with permission.)

activity within the amygdala and the ventromedial prefrontal cortex and strengthened connectivity between the amygdala and both the hippocampus and ventromedial prefrontal cortex during retrieval.[70] These findings are consistent with a study by Sterpenich and colleagues[71] and suggest that sleep strengthens the modulatory effect of the amygdala on other regions of the emotional memory network as memories undergo consolidation.[14] Whether these selective effects of sleep on emotional memory consolidation depend on REM sleep is an interesting question for future research.

BEYOND SLEEP STAGES

The above-mentioned results should not be taken to mean that SWS strictly mediates the consolidation of episodic memories, whereas REM sleep only mediates the consolidation of procedural and emotional memories. Matters are clearly not so simple. As mentioned in the previous sections, improvement on a visual discrimination task depends on SWS as well as REM,[24] and improvement on a motor task correlates with stage 2 NREM sleep.[29] Moreover, emotionally charged episodic memories may rely on both REM sleep and SWS for their consolidation.[7,72]

There are 2 possible interpretations of these apparent contradictions. First, the sleep stage dependency of these various memory tasks may depend on aspects of the task other than simply whether they are episodic or procedural, perhaps depending more on the intensity of training, the emotional salience of the task, or even the manner in which information is encoded (eg, deep vs shallow encoding or implicit vs explicit). The second possibility involves an inherent oversimplification in correlating performance improvements with sleep stages as they are classically defined. Indeed, mounting evidence points to several electrophysiological, neurotransmitter, and neuroendocrine mechanisms that may underlie these effects and that do not necessarily correlate with any single sleep stage, and sleep staging, as it has been defined for 40 years, may not capture all the key elements that lead to memory consolidation enhanced by sleep.

NEUROPHYSIOLOGICAL AND NEUROCHEMICAL EVIDENCE FOR SLEEP'S ROLE IN MEMORY CONSOLIDATION

Each of the above-mentioned sleep stages is characterized by a unique collection of electrophysiological, neurotransmitter, and neuroendocrine properties that tend to overlap with the different sleep stages but are not perfectly correlated with them. For example, SWS is associated with cortical slow oscillations (slow, <1 Hz oscillatory activity during SWS), sleep spindles (faster, 11–16 Hz, bursts of coherent brain activity), and hippocampal sharp wave-ripple complexes (approximately 200 Hz), all of which have been associated with episodic memory consolidation. Indeed, the co-occurrence of these electrophysiological events may underlie the coordinated information flow back and forth between the hippocampus and neocortex as memories are integrated within neocortical long-term storage sites.[13]

For example, slow oscillations are intensified when SWS is preceded by a learning experience[73–75] and hippocampus-dependent memories are specifically enhanced when slow oscillations are induced during SWS by transcranial electrical stimulation at 0.75 Hz (but not 5 Hz).[76]

Several human studies have shown a correlation between hippocampus-dependent episodic learning and cortical sleep spindles. In one such study,[77] subjects studied a long list of unrelated word pairs 1 hour before sleep, on 2 separate occasions at least a week apart. In one case, they were instructed to imagine a relationship between the 2 nominally unrelated words, whereas in the other they were simply asked to count the number of letters containing curved lines in each word pair. Such instructions lead to deep hippocampally mediated encoding and shallow cortically mediated encoding, respectively. During the subsequent nights of sleep, subjects showed significantly higher spindle densities on the nights after deep encoding, averaging 34% more spindles in the first 90 minutes of sleep. Moreover, sleep spindle density was positively correlated both with immediate recall tested in the final stage of training and with recall the next morning, after sleep. Thus, those who learned better had more spindles the following night and those with more spindles showed a greater performance gain the next morning.[78–80]

Hippocampal network oscillations such as sharp wave-ripple complexes may also help promote the synaptic plasticity necessary for memory consolidation. Such events can accompany the reactivation of hippocampal neuron ensembles that were activated during prior waking training. Moreover, inducing long-term potentiation, a neurophysiological mechanism of learning and memory, can trigger the generation of sharp wave-ripple complexes in the rat hippocampus,[81] suggesting that strengthened synaptic coupling can lead to neurons firing synchronously during formation of sharp wave-ripples complexes. Connecting these events to behavior, Eschenko and colleagues[82] demonstrated that rats learning odor-reward associations produced an increase in the number and size of ripple events for 2 hours during subsequent SWS. Moreover, episodic memory consolidation in human epileptic patients correlates with the number of ripples recorded from the major output regions of the hippocampus (perirhinal and entorhinal cortices),[83] and selective disruption of hippocampal ripples by electric stimulation during postlearning rest phases in rats impairs formation of long-lasting spatial memories, suggesting that ripples could have a causal role in sleep-based memory consolidation.[84]

Recent work also suggests that there is a close temporal relationship between the occurrence of slow oscillations, spindles, and sharp wave-ripple complexes during SWS that may coordinate bidirectional information flow between the hippocampus and neocortex as memories are integrated within long-term storage sites.

NEUROTRANSMITTERS AND NEUROHORMONES

There is also evidence to suggest that nocturnal changes in neurotransmitter and neurohormone levels contribute to memory consolidation. ACh, norepinephrine, 5-HT, and cortisol play important roles both in modulating sleep[85] and memory function.[86–88] Cortisol levels, for instance, follow a marked circadian rhythm, whereby the hormone is at its nadir during early-night slow wave–rich sleep and reaches its zenith during late-night REM-rich sleep. Indeed, the difference between the cortisol level in the blood at sleep onset and at awakening is so great that the interpretation of cortisol blood levels is meaningless without knowing exactly when the sample was taken.[89–91] Moreover, the secretion of cortisol is not continuous but composed of gradually increasing peaks that tend to coincide with REM sleep (**Fig. 8**). REM sleep thus tends to co-occur with cortisol elevations.[90,92]

The early night reduction in ACh and cortisol levels may be necessary for hippocampus-dependent memories to undergo effective consolidation because experimentally elevating the levels of either substance during early sleep impairs performance on episodic memory tasks. Gais and Born[93] trained subjects on word pair task and mirror tracing tasks before 3 hours of nocturnal sleep or wakefulness during which they received a placebo or an infusion of the cholinesterase inhibitor physostigmine (which increases cholinergic tone). When tested after 3 hours of early sleep rich in SWS, recall on the paired associates task was markedly impaired in the physostigmine group, while the procedural memory performance was unaffected. Using a similar design, Plihal and Born[94] showed that when cortisol was infused during the early SWS-rich interval, retention of episodic information that is

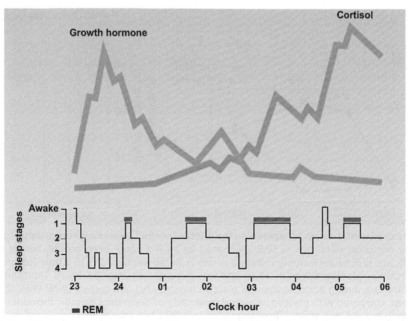

Fig. 8. The relationship between sleep stage architecture and circulating levels of growth hormone and cortisol. Note both the linear increase in cortisol levels across the night and also the cortisol peaks riding on top of the REM periods.

normally facilitated during this time was impaired. Thus, enhancing plasma cortisol concentrations during early sleep eradicated the benefit typically observed for episodic memory while leaving procedural memory unimpaired (**Fig. 9**).

Plihal and Born[94] concluded that because episodic, but not procedural, memory relies on hippocampal function, cortisol inhibition during early nocturnal sleep is necessary for episodic memory consolidation. Thus, because cortisol release is normally inhibited during early night periods dense in SWS, this time window may provide the ideal physiologic environment for episodic memory consolidation. REM sleep, on the other hand, is an inefficient time to consolidate episodes because of the deleterious effect of elevated cortisol on hippocampus-dependent memory processing. Thus, the neurobiological properties of early sleep and late sleep, as opposed to SWS and REM sleep per se, may be essential for the consolidation of different types of memory.

In line with the above-mentioned findings, elevation of cortisol levels during wakefulness can also impair performance on episodic memory.[89,95] The cortisol level in the Plihal and Born[94] study (15.2 + 0.68 mg/dL) was elevated just enough to mimic the late night peak of circadian cortisol activity and is proportionate to the amount of cortisol typically released in response to a mild to moderate stressor (approximately 10–30 mg/dL) and is a sufficient dose to disrupt episodic memory function during wakefulness,[89,92,96,97] particularly when administered prior to consolidation or at

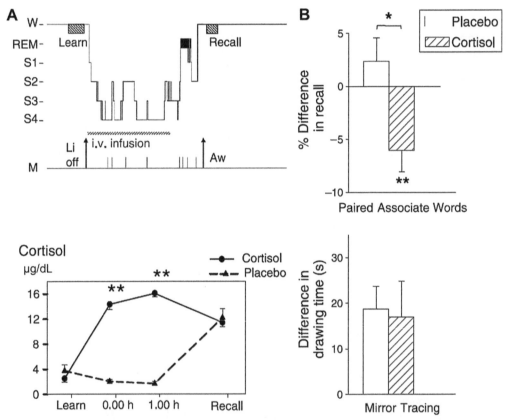

Fig. 9. (*A, top*) Experimental design for examining the effect of cortisol on memory consolidation during a 3-hour period of early nocturnal sleep rich in SWS, illustrated by an individual sleep profile. Before sleep, subjects learned episodic and procedural memory tasks to a criterion. Recall was tested 15 to 30 minutes after awakening. Infusion of cortisol or placebo began at 11 PM and was discontinued after 2.5 hours. (*Bottom*) Mean plasma cortisol concentrations during administration of placebo (*dotted line*) and cortisol (*solid line*). (*B*) Cortisol infusion during sleep, compared with placebo, impaired hippocampus-dependent episodic memories for word pairs across sleep (*top*), but did not affect hippocampus-independent procedural memory (speed in mirror tracing, *bottom*). N = 14, *$P<.05$, **$P<.01$. Aw, awake; IV, intravenous, Li, lights; S, stage; W, wake. (*Data from* Plihal W, Born J. Memory consolidation in human sleep depends on inhibition of glucocorticoid release. Neuroreport 1999;10(13):2741–7.)

retrieval.[95,98] Elevations in cortisol levels seen during late night REM sleep may help explain why replay of episodic memories in REM sleep dreaming is so scarce[99] and perhaps also why dreams are difficult to remember on awakening.[87,100]

In addition to cortisol, other hormones (eg, growth hormone) are also known to affect memory function in the waking state and vary across sleep, suggesting that they might modulate sleep-based memory consolidation as well. Although initial studies of growth hormone have failed to find such an effect,[101] further investigation of the neurochemistry underlying the relationship between sleep and memory consolidation is a productive avenue for future research. Indeed, it seems especially important to forge ahead into precisely this neuromodulatory realm, in which the chemical basis of the sleep/memory consolidation connection can be examined.

FUTURE DIRECTIONS

Over the past 10 years, the field of sleep and memory has grown exponentially, with reports of sleep-memory interactions emerging from myriad disciplines and ranging from cellular and molecular studies in animals to behavioral and neuroimaging studies in humans. Correspondingly little is known, however, about sleep-dependent memory consolidation in diverse clinical conditions that are associated with sleep impairment. These conditions range from physical conditions, such as sleep apnea, to psychiatric conditions, such as depression, and each condition may affect sleep-dependent memory processing in profound but different ways.

For example, obstructive sleep apnea (OSA) is characterized by repetitive breathing cessations during sleep that can produce hundreds of short EEG arousals each night. Although the cognitive deficits associated with OSA are well documented[102] and the hypoxia associated with OSA is thought to alter brain regions (eg, hippocampus) that underlie the cognitive deficits,[103,104] very little research has directly assessed decrements to sleep-dependent memory consolidation in this population (see[105] for a notable exception). Similarly, depression and schizophrenia, both of which are associated with marked changes in sleep architecture,[106] have recently been associated with disrupted procedural memory consolidation,[48,49] yet a careful study of sleep-related episodic, and especially emotional, memory consolidation in these populations have yet to be conducted. These are but 3 examples of the vital and potentially fruitful questions that remain to be answered about sleep-dependent memory consolidation in the clinical realm. Future research in the field should thus target clinical conditions that are characterized by sleep deficits, assessing to what degree sleep dysfunction is associated with impaired memory consolidation, and, equally importantly, determining whether sleep treatment will yield cognitive, emotional, and physical benefits.

REFERENCES

1. Hobson JA, McCarley RW, Wyzinski PW. Sleep cycle oscillation: reciprocal discharge by two brainstem neuronal groups. Science 1975;189: 55–8.
2. Walker MP, Stickgold R. Sleep, memory and plasticity. Annu Rev Psychol 2006;57:139–66.
3. Stickgold R, Hobson JA, Fosse R. Sleep, learning, and dreams: off-line memory reprocessing. Science 2001;294:1052–7.
4. McGaugh JL. Memory – a century of consolidation. Science 2000;287:248–51.
5. Diekelmann S, Born J. The memory function of sleep. Nat Rev Neurosci 2010;11:114–26.
6. Payne JD, Ellenbogen JM, Walker MP, et al. The role of sleep in memory consolidation. In: Byrne JH, editor. Concise learning and memory: the editor's selection. Oxford (UK): Elsevier Press; 2008. p. 547–69.
7. Payne JD, Kensinger EA. Sleep's role in the consolidation of emotional episodic memories. Curr Dir Psychol Sci 2010;19(5):290–5.
8. Stickgold R. Sleep-dependent memory consolidation. Nature 2005;437:1272–8.
9. Smith C. Sleep states, memory processes and synaptic plasticity. Behav Brain Res 1995;78: 49–56.
10. Walker MP. The role of sleep in cognition and emotion. Ann N Y Acad Sci 2009;1156:168–97.
11. Schacter DL, Tulving E. Memory systems 1994. Cambridge (MA): MIT Press; 1994.
12. Hamann SB. Cognitive and neural mechanisms of emotional memory. Trends Cogn Sci 2001;5: 394–400.
13. Moscovitch M, Rosenbaum RS, Gilboa A, et al. Functional neuroanatomy of remote episodic, semantic and spatial memory: a unified account based on multiple trace theory. J Anat 2005; 207(1):35–66.
14. McGaugh JL. The amygdala modulates the consolidation of memories of emotionally arousing experiences. Annu Rev Neurosci 2004;27:1–28.
15. Giuditta A, Ambrosini MV, Montagnese P, et al. The sequential hypothesis of the function of sleep. Behav Brain Res 1995;69:157–66.

16. Marshall L, Born J. The contribution of sleep to hippocampus-dependent memory consolidation. Trends Cogn Sci 2007;11:442–50.

17. Nishida M, Pearsall J, Buckner RL, et al. REM sleep, prefrontal theta and the consolidation of human emotional memory. Cereb Cortex 2009;19:1158–66.

18. Walker MP, Stickgold R. Overnight alchemy: sleep-dependent memory evolution. Nat Rev Neurosci 2010;11:218.

19. Karni A, Sagi D. The time course of learning a visual skill. Nature 1993;365:250–2.

20. Karni A, Tanne D, Rubenstein BS, et al. Dependence on REM sleep of overnight improvement of a perceptual skill. Science 1994;265(5172):679–82.

21. Stickgold R. Human studies of sleep and off-line memory reprocessing. In: Maquet P, Smith C, Stickgold R, editors. Sleep and plasticity. London: Oxford University Press; 2003. p. 41–65.

22. Stickgold R, James L, Hobson JA. Visual discrimination learning requires post-training sleep. Nat Neurosci 2000;2(12):1237–8.

23. Stickgold R, Whidbee D, Schirmer B, et al. Visual discrimination task improvement: a multi-step process occurring during sleep. J Cogn Neurosci 2000;12:246–54.

24. Gais S, Plihal W, Wagner U, et al. Early sleep triggers memory for early visual discrimination skills. Nat Neurosci 2000;3(12):1335–9.

25. Mednick S, Nakayama K, Stickgold R. Sleep dependent learning: a nap is as good as a night. Nat Neurosci 2003;6:697–8.

26. Mednick SC, Nakayama K, Cantero JL, et al. The restorative effect of naps on perceptual deterioration. Nat Neurosci 2002;5:677–81.

27. Walker M, Brakefield T, Morgan A, et al. Practice with sleep makes perfect: sleep dependent motor skill learning. Neuron 2002;35:205–11.

28. Fogel S, Jacob J, Smith C. Increased sleep spindle activity following simple motor procedural learning in humans. Actas de Fisiología 2001;7:123.

29. Smith C, MacNeill C. Impaired motor memory for a pursuit rotor task following Stage 2 sleep loss in college students. J Sleep Res 1994;3:206–13.

30. Tweed S, Aubrey JB, Nader R, et al. Deprivation of REM sleep or stage 2 sleep differentially affects cognitive procedural and motor procedural memory. Sleep 1999;22:S241.

31. Sejnowski TJ, Destexhe A. Why do we sleep? Brain Res 2000;886(1–2):208–23.

32. Kuriyama K, Stickgold R, Walker MP. Sleep-dependent learning and motor-skill complexity. Learn Mem 2004;11(6):705–13.

33. Maquet P, Laureys S, Perrin F, et al. Festina lente: evidences for fast and slow learning processes and a role for sleep in human motor skill learning. Learn Mem 2003;10(4):237–9.

34. Hennevin E, Hars B, Maho C, et al. Processing of learned information in paradoxical sleep: relevance for memory. Behav Brain Res 1995;69:125–35.

35. Smith C, Wong PT. Paradoxical sleep increases predict successful learning in a complex operant task. Behav Neurosci 1991;105(2):282–8.

36. Smith C, Young J, Young W. Prolonged increases in paradoxical sleep during and after avoidance-task acquisition. Sleep 1980;3(1):67–81.

37. Maquet P, Laureys S, Peigneux P, et al. Experience-dependent changes in cerebral activation during human REM sleep. Nat Neurosci 2000;3(8):831–6.

38. Peigneux P, Laureys S, Fuchs S, et al. Learned material content and acquisition level modulate cerebral reactivation during posttraining rapid-eye-movements sleep. Neuroimage 2003;20(1):125–34.

39. Datta S. Avoidance task training potentiates phasic pontine-wave density in the rat: a mechanism for sleep-dependent plasticity. J Neurosci 2000;20(22):8607–13.

40. Datta S, Mavanji V, Ulloor J, et al. Activation of phasic pontine-wave generator prevents rapid eye movement sleep deprivation-induced learning impairment in the rat: a mechanism for sleep-dependent plasticity. J Neurosci 2004;24(6):1416–27.

41. Smith C. Sleep states and memory processes in humans: procedural versus declarative memory systems. Sleep Med Rev 2001;5(6):491–506.

42. Greenberg R, Pearlman CA. Cutting the REM nerve: an approach to the adaptive function of REM sleep. Perspect Biol Med 1974;17:513–21.

43. Robertson EM, Cohen DA. Understanding consolidation through the architecture of memories. Neuroscientist 2006;12:261–71.

44. Robertson EM, Pascual-Leone A, Press DZ. Awareness modifies the skill-learning benefits of sleep. Curr Biol 2004;14:208–12.

45. Nissen C, Kloepfer C, Nofzinger EA, et al. Impaired sleep-related memory consolidation in primary insomnia – a pilot study. Sleep 2006;29:1068–73.

46. Manoach D, Thakkar KN, Stroynowski E, et al. Reduced overnight consolidation of procedural learning in chronic medicated schizophrenia is related to specific sleep stages. J Psychiatr Res 2009;44(2):112–20.

47. Maquet P. The role of sleep in learning and memory. Science 2001;294(5544):1048–52.

48. Manoach DS, Cain MS, Vangel MG, et al. A failure of sleep-dependent procedural learning in chronic, medicated schizophrenia. Biol Psychiatry 2004;56:951–6.

49. Dresler M, Kluge M, Genzel L, et al. Impaired off-line memory consolidation in depression. Eur Neuropsychopharmacol 2010;20:533–61.

50. Plihal W, Born J. Effects of early and late nocturnal sleep on declarative and procedural memory. J Cogn Neurosci 1997;9(4):534–47.

51. Tucker MA, Hirota Y, Wamsley EJ, et al. A daytime nap containing solely non-REM sleep enhances declarative but not procedural memory. Neurobiol Learn Mem 2006;86(2):241–7.

52. Ji D, Wilson MA. Coordinated memory replay in the visual cortex and hippocampus during sleep. Nat Neurosci 2007;10:100–7.

53. Wilson MA, McNaughton BL. Reactivation of hippocampal ensemble memories during sleep. Science 1994;265:676–9.

54. O'Neil J, Pleydell-Bouverie B, Dupret D, et al. Play it again: reactivation of waking experience and memory. Trends Neurosci 2010;33(5):220–9.

55. Peigneux P, Laureys S, Fuchs S, et al. Are spatial memories strengthened in the human hippocampus during slow wave sleep? Neuron 2004; 44:535–45.

56. Rasch B, Buchel C, Gias S, et al. Odor cues during slow-wave sleep prompt declarative memory consolidation. Science 2007;315:1426–9.

57. Takashima A, Petersson KM, Rutters F, et al. Declarative memory consolidation in humans: a prospective functional magnetic resonance imaging study. Proc Natl Acad Sci U S A 2006; 103(3):756–61.

58. Hu P, Stylos-Allan M, Walker M. Sleep facilitates consolidation of emotional declarative memory. Psychol Sci 2006;17:891–8.

59. Wagner U, Gais S, Born J. Emotional memory formation is enhanced across sleep intervals with high amounts of rapid eye movement sleep. Learn Mem 2001;8:112–9.

60. Wagner U, Hallschmid M, Rasch B, et al. Brief sleep after learning keeps emotional memories alive for years. Biol Psychiatry 2006;60:788–90.

61. Maquet P, Péters JM, Aerts J, et al. Functional neuroanatomy of human rapid-eye-movement sleep and dreaming. Nature 1996;383:163–6.

62. Greenberg R, Pearlman C, Schwartz W, et al. Memory, emotion, and REM sleep. J Abnorm Psychol 1983;92:378–81.

63. Ellenbogen JM, Payne JD, Stickgold R. Sleep's role in declarative memory consolidation: passive, permissive, active or none? Curr Opin Neurobiol 2006;16:716–22.

64. Bartlett FC. Remembering: a study in experimental and social psychology. Cambridge (UK): Cambridge University Press; 1932.

65. Ellenbogen JM, Hu P, Payne JD, et al. Human relational memory requires time and sleep. Proc Natl Acad Sci U S A 2007;104:7723–8.

66. Schacter DL, Addis DR, Buckner RL. Episodic simulation of future events. Ann N Y Acad Sci 2008;1124:39–60.

67. Payne JD, Stickgold R, Swanberg K, et al. Sleep preferentially enhances memory for emotional components of scenes. Psychol Sci 2008;19:781–8.

68. Payne JD, Schacter DL, Tucker MA, et al. The role of sleep in false memory formation. Neurobiol Learn Mem 2009;92:327–34.

69. Wagner U, Gais S, Haider H, et al. Sleep inspires insight. Nature 2004;427:352–5.

70. Payne JD, Kensinger EA. Sleep leads to qualitative changes in the emotional memory trace: evidence from fMRI. J Cogn Neurosci 2010. DOI:10.1162/jocn.2010.21526.

71. Sterpenich V, Albouy G, Darsaud A, et al. Sleep promotes the neural reorganization of remote emotional memory. J Neurosci 2009;29:5143–52.

72. Payne JD, Nadel L. Sleep, dreams, and memory consolidation: the role of the stress hormone cortisol. Learn Mem 2004;11:671–8.

73. Huber R, Ghilardi MF, Massimini M, et al. Local sleep and learning. Nature 2004;430:78–81.

74. Molle M, Marshall L, Gais S, et al. Learning increases human electroencephalographic coherence during subsequent slow sleep oscillations. Proc Natl Acad Sci U S A 2004;101:13963–8.

75. Molle M, Eschenko O, Gais S, et al. The influence of learning on sleep slow oscillations and associated spindles and ripples in humans and rats. Eur J Neurosci 2009;29:1071–81.

76. Marshall L, Helgadottir H, Molle M, et al. Boosting slow oscillations during sleep potentiates memory. Nature 2006;444:610–3.

77. Gais S, Molle M, Helms K, et al. Learning-dependent increases in sleep spindle density. J Neurosci 2002;22(15):6830–4.

78. Schmidt C, Peigneux P, Muto V, et al. Encoding difficulty promotes postlearning changes in sleep spindle activity during napping. J Neurosci 2006; 26:8976–82.

79. Clemens Z, Fabo D, Halasz P. Twenty-four hours retention of visuospatial memory correlates with the number of parietal sleep spindles. Neurosci Lett 2006;403:52–6.

80. Schabus M, Hodlmoser K, Gruber G, et al. Sleep spindle-related activity in the human EEG and its relation to general cognitive and learning abilities. Eur J Neurosci 2006;23(7):1738–46.

81. Behrens CJ, van den Boom LP, et al. Induction of sharp wave-ripple complexes in vitro and reorganization of hippocampal networks. Nat Neurosci 2005;8:1560–7.

82. Eschenko O, Ramadan W, Molle M, et al. Sustained increase in hippocampal sharp-wave ripple activity during slow-wave sleep after learning. Learn Mem 2008;15:222–8.

83. Axmacher N, Elger CE, Fell J. Ripples in the medial temporal lobe are relevant for human memory consolidation. Brain 2008;131:1806–17.

84. Girardeau G, Benchenane K, Wiener SI, et al. Selective suppression of hippocampal ripples impairs spatial memory. Nat Neurosci 2009;12: 1222–3.

85. Hobson JA, Pace-Schott EF. The cognitive neuroscience of sleep: neuronal systems, consciousness and learning. Nat Rev Neurosci 2002;3: 679–93.

86. Cahill L, McGaugh JL. Mechanisms of emotional arousal and lasting declarative memory. Trends Neurosci 1998;21:294–9.

87. Payne JD. Memory consolidation, the diurnal rhythm of cortisol, and the nature of dreams: a new hypothesis. Int Rev Neurobiol 2010;92: 101–36.

88. Hasselmo ME. Neuromodulation: acetylcholine and memory consolidation. Trends Cogn Sci 1999;3: 351–9.

89. Payne JD, Nadel L, Britton WB, et al. The biopsychology of trauma and memory. In: Reisberg D, Hertel P, editors. Emotion and memory. Oxford (UK): Oxford University Press; 2004. p. 76–127.

90. Lavie P. The enchanted world of sleep. New Haven (CT): Yale University Press; 1996.

91. Weitzman ED, Fukushima D, Nogeire C, et al. Twenty-four hour pattern of the episodic secretion of cortisol in normal subjects. J Clin Endocrinol Metab 1971;33:14–22.

92. Wagner U, Born J. Memory consolidation during sleep: interactive effects of sleep stages and HPA regulation. Stress 2008;11:28–41.

93. Gais S, Born J. Low acetylcholine during slow-wave sleep is critical for declarative memory consolidation. Proc Natl Acad Sci U S A 2004; 101(7):2140–4.

94. Plihal W, Born J. Memory consolidation in human sleep depends on inhibition of glucocorticoid release. Neuroreport 1999;10(13):2741–7.

95. de Quervain DJF, Aerni A, Schelling G, et al. Glucocorticoids and the regulation of memory in health and disease. Front Neuroendocrinol 2009; 30:358–70.

96. Kirschbaum C, Wolf OT, May M, et al. Stress and treatment induced elevations of cortisol levels associated with impaired declarative memory in healthy adults. Life Sci 1996;58:1475–83.

97. Kirschbaum C, Pirke K, Hellhammer D. The 'Trier Social Stress Test' - A tool for investigating psychobiological stress responses in a laboratory setting. Neuropsychobiology 1993;28:76–81.

98. de Quervain DJF, Roozendaal B, Nitsch RM, et al. Acute cortisone administration impairs retrieval of long-term declarative memory in humans. Nat Neurosci 2000;3:313–4.

99. Fosse MJ, Fosse R, Hobson JA, et al. Dreaming and episodic memory: a functional dissociation? J Cogn Neurosci 2003;15:1–9.

100. Hobson JA. The dreaming brain. New York: Basic Books; 1988.

101. Gais S, Hullemann P, Hallschmid M, et al. Sleep-dependent surges in growth hormones do not contribute to sleep-dependent memory consolidation. Psychoneuroendocrinology 2006;31(6):786–91.

102. Saunamaki T, Jehkonen M. A review of executive functions in obstructive sleep apnea syndrome. Acta Neurol Scand 2007;115:1–11.

103. Meerlo P, Mistlberger RE, Jacobs BL, et al. New neurons in the adult brain: the role of sleep and consequences of sleep loss. Sleep Med Rev 2009;13:187–94.

104. Row BW. Intermittent hypoxia and cognitive function: implications from chronic animal models. Adv Exp Med Biol 2007;618:51–67.

105. Kloepfer C, Riemann D, Nofzinger EA, et al. Memory before and after sleep in patients with moderate obstructive sleep apnea. J Clin Sleep Med 2009;5:540–8.

106. Armitage R. Sleep and circadian rhythms in mood disorders. Acta Psychiatr Scand 2007; 115(Suppl 433):104–15.

Sleep and Emotional Memory Processing

Els van der Helm, MSc, Matthew P. Walker, PhD[*]

KEYWORDS

- Sleep • REM sleep • Emotion • Affect • Learning • Memory
- Depression • PTSD

The ability of the human brain to generate, regulate, and be guided by emotions represents a fundamental process governing not only our personal lives but also our mental health and societal structure. The recent emergence of cognitive neuroscience has ushered in a new era of research connecting affective behavior with human brain function and has provided a systems-level view of emotional information processing, translationally bridging animal models of affective regulation and relevant clinical disorders.[1,2]

Independent of this research area, a recent resurgence has also taken place within the basic sciences, focusing on the functional effect of sleep on neurocognitive processes.[3] However, surprisingly less research attention has been given to the interaction between sleep and affective brain function, considering the remarkable overlap between the known physiology of sleep, especially rapid eye movement (REM) sleep, and the associated neurochemistry and network anatomy that modulate emotions, as well as the prominent co-occurrence of abnormal sleep (including REM sleep) in almost all affective psychiatric and mood disorders.

Despite the relative historical paucity of research, recent work has begun to describe a consistent and clarifying role of sleep in the selective modulation of emotional memory and affective regulation. This review provides a synthesis of these findings, describing an intimate relationship between sleep, emotional brain function, and clinical mood disorders and offers a tentative first theoretical framework that may account for these observed interactions.

SLEEP

The sleep of mammalian species has been broadly classified into 2 distinct types; non-REM (NREM) sleep and REM sleep, with NREM sleep being further divided in primates and cats into 4 substages (1–4) corresponding, in that order, to increasing depth of sleep.[4] In humans, NREM and REM sleep alternate or "cycle" across the night in an ultradian pattern every 90 minutes (**Fig. 1**). Although this NREM-REM cycle length remains largely stable across the night, the ratio of NREM to REM within each 90-minute cycle changes, so that early in the night, stages 3 and 4 of NREM dominate, whereas stage-2 NREM and REM sleep prevail in the latter half of the night. The functional reasons for this organizing principal (deep NREM early in the night, stage-2 NREM and REM late in the night) remain unknown.[5]

As NREM sleep progresses, electroencephalographic (EEG) activity begins to slow in frequency. Throughout stage-2 NREM, there is the presence of phasic electrical events, including K-complexes (large electrical sharp waves in the EEG) and sleep spindles (short synchronized bursts of EEG electrical activity in the 11–15 Hz range).[6] The deepest stages of NREM, stages 3 and 4, are often grouped together under the term slow wave sleep (SWS), reflecting the occurrence of low frequency waves (0.5–4 Hz), representing an expression of underlying mass cortical synchrony.[7,8] During REM sleep, however, EEG wave forms once again change in their composition, associated with oscillatory activity in the theta band range (4–7 Hz),

Sleep and Neuroimaging Laboratory, Department of Psychology and Helen Wills Neuroscience Institute, University of California, 3331 Tolman Hall, Berkeley, CA 94720-1650, USA
* Corresponding author. Department of Psychology, University of California, 3331 Tolman Hall, Berkeley, CA 94720-1650.
E-mail address: mpwalker@berkeley.edu

Sleep Med Clin 6 (2011) 31–43
doi:10.1016/j.jsmc.2010.12.010

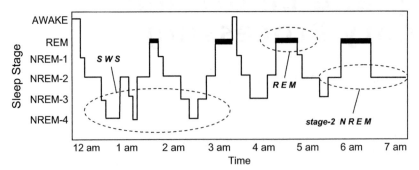

Fig. 1. The human sleep cycle. Across the night, NREM and REM sleep cycle every 90 minutes in an ultradian manner, while the ratio of NREM to REM sleep shifts. During the first half of the night, NREM stages 3 and 4 NREM (SWS) dominate, while stage-2 NREM and REM sleep prevail in the latter half of the night. EEG patterns also differ significantly between sleep stages, with electrical oscillations, such as slow delta waves developing in SWS, K-complexes and sleep spindles occurring during stage-2 NREM, and theta waves seen during REM.

together with higher frequency synchronous activity in the 30 to 80 Hz (gamma) range.[9,10] Periodic bursts of rapid eye movement also take place, a defining characteristic of REM sleep, associated with the occurrence of phasic endogenous waveforms. These waveforms are expressed in, among other regions, the pons (P), lateral geniculate nuclei of the thalamus (G), and the occipital cortex (O), and as such, have been termed PGO waves.[11]

As the brain passes through these sleep stages, it also undergoes dramatic alterations in neurochemistry.[12] In NREM sleep, subcortical cholinergic systems in the brainstem and forebrain become markedly less active[13,14] while firing rates of serotonergic Raphé neurons and noradrenergic locus coeruleus neurons are also reduced relative to waking levels.[15,16] During REM sleep, both these aminergic populations are strongly inhibited, while the cholinergic systems become as or more active compared with wake,[17,18] resulting in a brain state largely devoid of aminergic modulation and dominated by acetylcholine (ACh).

At a whole-brain systems level, neuroimaging techniques have revealed complex and dramatically different patterns of functional anatomy associated with NREM and REM sleep (for review, see[19]). During NREM SWS, brainstem, thalamic, basal ganglia, prefrontal, and temporal lobe regions all appear to undergo reduced activity. However, during REM sleep, significant elevations in levels of activity have been reported in the pontine tegmentum, thalamic nuclei, occipital cortex, mediobasal prefrontal lobes together with affect-related regions including the amygdala, hippocampus, and anterior cingulate cortex **(Fig. 2)**. In contrast, the dorsolateral prefrontal cortex, posterior cingulate, and parietal cortex appear least active in REM sleep.

Although this summary only begins to describe the range of neural processes that are affected by the brain's daily transit through sleep states, it clearly demonstrates that sleep itself cannot be treated as a homogeneous entity, offering a range of distinct neurobiological mechanisms that can support numerous brain functions. The following sections examine the role of sleep, and specific stages of sleep, in the modulation of emotional memories and the regulation of affective reactivity, which culminate in a heuristic model of sleep-dependent emotional brain processing.

Sleep and Emotional Memory Processing

The effect of sleep has principally been characterized at 2 different stages of memory: (1) before learning, in the initial formation (encoding) of new information; and (2) after learning, in the long-term solidification (consolidation) of new memories.[3,20,21] Each of these stages are considered now, and focus is on reports involving affective learning.

Sleep and Affective Memory Encoding

The initial stage of memory formation can be strongly modulated by the elicitation of emotion at the time of learning.[22] Emotionally arousing stimuli are consistently remembered better than neutral stimuli both in experimental laboratory studies and in real-life accounts (Heuer and Reisberg 1990[23]; Bradley and colleagues 1992[24]; Buchanan and Lovallo 2001[25]; Christianson, 1992[26]); studies of autobiographical memory have found that individuals are more likely to remember those events that have increased emotional and personal significance.[27] The adrenergic system appears to play a key role in orchestrating the enhancing effect of arousing emotion on memory at the initial moment of learning (and

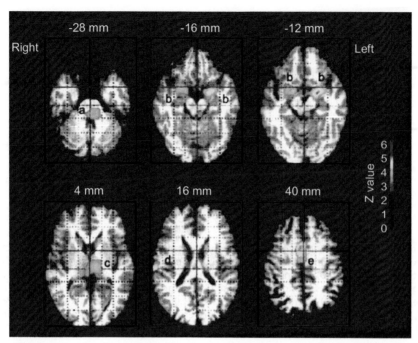

Fig. 2. Regional brain activation during REM sleep (positron emission tomography scan). The areas include: (a) the pons; (b) amygdala; (c) thalamus; (d) right parietal operculum; and (e) anterior cingulate cortex. The z-value color scale indicates strength of activation. A z value of 3.09 corresponds to a P value of less than .001. (*Data from* Maquet P, Peters JM, Aerts J, et al. Functional neuroanatomy of human rapid-eye-movement sleep and dreaming. Nature 1996;383:163.)

also during consolidation, discussed later). For example, Cahill and colleagues[28] have demonstrated that the administration of propanolol, a β-adrenoceptor antagonist, to participants before learning of emotional and neutral narrative texts blocks the memory enhancing effects elicited by arousal. Similarly, propranolol administration before the encoding of affectively arousing word stimuli subverts the normal facilitation of emotional memory recall when tested shortly after.[29] However, this autonomic enhancing effect on memory is not observed in patients with amygdala lesions, suggesting a role not only for a specific neurochemical system in affective learning but also for a particular brain region.[30,31] Indeed, functional neuroimaging studies have since confirmed the critical role of the amygdala in facilitating emotional memory formation at the time of experience.[28–36]

These beneficial enhancing effects of emotion on the initial process of learning pertain to conditions when the brain has obtained adequate prior sleep. There is now considerable evidence that sleep loss before encoding can significantly and selectively alter and impair the canonical profile of emotional memory enhancement. Although early studies investigating the role of sleep-dependent memory in humans focused primarily on postlearning consolidation (see later sections),

more recent data similarly support the need for adequate prelearning sleep in the formation of new human episodic memories. Some of the first studies of sleep deprivation and memory encoding focused on neutral forms of learning, indicating that the temporal memory (ie, the memory for events that occur) was significantly disrupted by a night of pretraining sleep deprivation[37,38]; even when caffeine was administered to overcome nonspecific effects of lower arousal.

More recent investigations have examined the importance of pretraining sleep for the formation of emotional and neutral memories.[3] Subjects were either sleep deprived for 36 hours or allowed to sleep normally before a learning session composed of emotionally negative, positive, and neutral words, with the efficiency of encoding subsequently tested after 2 recovery nights of sleep. Averaged across all memory categories, subjects who were sleep deprived demonstrated a 40% deficit in memory encoding, relative to subjects who had slept normally before learning (**Fig. 3**A). However, when these data were separated into the 3 emotional categories (negative, positive, or neutral), selective dissociations became apparent (see **Fig. 3**B). In subjects who had slept (control group), both positive and negative stimuli were associated with superior retention levels relative to the neutral condition,

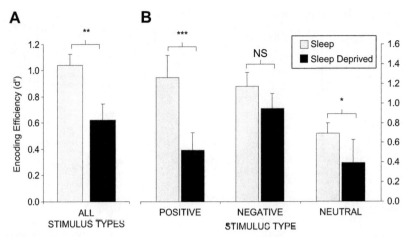

Fig. 3. Sleep deprivation and encoding of emotional and nonemotional declarative memory. Effects of 38 hours of total sleep deprivation on encoding of human declarative memory. (*A*) When combined across all emotional and nonemotional categories. (*B*) When separated by emotional (positive and negative valence) and nonemotional (neutral valence) categories, demonstrating a significant group (sleep, sleep-deprivation) × emotion category (positive, negative, neutral) interaction ($F[1,18]$ 3.58, $P<.05$). Post hoc t-test comparisons: *$P<.08$, **$P<.05$, ***$P<.01$; NS, not significant; error bars represent standard error of the mean. d′, d-prime (discrimination index). (*From* Walker MP, Stickgold R. Sleep, memory, and plasticity. Annu Rev Psychol 2006;57:139–66; Fig. 2, p. 144; with permission.)

consistent with the notion that emotion facilitates memory encoding.[22] In the sleep-deprived group, a severe encoding impairment was evident for neutral and especially positive emotional memories, showing a significant 59% retention deficit, relative to the control condition. Most interesting was the relative resistance of negative emotional memory to sleep deprivation, showing a markedly smaller and nonsignificant impairment.

These data indicate that sleep loss impairs the ability to commit new experiences to memory and has recently been associated with dysfunction throughout the hippocampal complex.[39] The data also suggest that, although the effects of sleep deprivation are directionally consistent across emotional subcategories, the most profound effect is on the encoding of positive emotional stimuli, and to a lesser degree, on the emotionally neutral stimuli. In contrast, the encoding of negative memory seems to be more resistant to the effects of prior sleep loss. Moreover, such results may offer novel learning and memory insights into affective mood disorders that express co-occurring sleep abnormalities,[40] whereby sleep deprivation imposes a skewed distribution of learning, resulting in a dominance of negative memory representations.

Sleep and Affective Memory Consolidation

The role of sleep in declarative memory consolidation, rather than being absolute, may depend on more intricate aspects of the information being learned, such as the novelty, the meaning to extract, and also the affective salience of the material. A collection of findings has described a preferential offline consolidation benefit (reduction in forgetting) for emotional information compared with neutral information. Furthermore, this differential emotional advantage seems to persist and even improve over periods containing a night of sleep.[36,41–44] Indeed, several reports have directly examined whether it is time, with sleep, that preferentially modulates these effects. Based on the coincident neurophysiology that REM sleep provides and the neurobiological requirements of emotional memory processing,[45,46] work has now begun to test a selective REM sleep-dependent hypothesis of affective human memory consolidation.

For example, Hu and colleagues[47] have compared the consolidation of emotionally arousing and nonarousing picture stimuli after a 12-hour period across a day or after a night of sleep. A specific emotional memory benefit was observed only after sleep and not across an equivalent time awake. Atienza and Cantero[15] have also demonstrated that total sleep deprivation the first night after learning significantly impairs later 1-week retention of emotional as well as neutral visual stimuli. This difference was greatest for neutral items relative to emotional items. Such a difference may indicate that emotional items are more resistant to the effect of first-night sleep deprivation (a finding with clinical treatment consequences), or that subsequent postdeprivation recovery sleep is more capable of salvaging consolidation of emotional relative to neutral memories. Wagner and colleagues[48] have also shown that sleep selectively favors the retention of previously learned emotional texts relative to neutral texts, and that this affective memory benefit is only present after late-night sleep (a period rich in REM sleep). This emotional memory benefit was found to persist in a follow-up study performed 4 years later.[49] It has also been demonstrated that the speed of recognizing emotional face expressions presented before sleep is significantly improved the next day, a benefit that is positively correlated with the amount of intervening REM sleep.[50]

Sleep has also been shown to target the consolidation of specific aspects of emotional experiences, as well as mediate the extinction of human fear memories. By experimentally varying the foreground and background elements of emotional picture stimuli, Payne and colleagues[51] have demonstrated that sleep can target the strengthening of negative emotional objects in a scene but not in the peripheral background. In contrast, equivalent time awake did not afford any selective benefit to emotional object memory (or the background scene). This finding may suggest that sleep-dependent processing can selectively separate episodic experience into component parts, preferentially consolidating those of greatest affective salience. Using a conditioning paradigm in humans, Pace-Schott and colleagues[52] recently investigated the effects of sleep and wake on fear extinction and generalization of fear extinction. Concurrent fear conditioning to 2 different stimuli was followed by targeted extinction of conditioned responding to only 1 of the stimuli. Participants were then tested after a 12-hour offline delay period across the day or after a night of sleep. On returning 12 hours later, generalization of extinction from the target stimuli to the nontargeted stimuli occurred after a night of sleep, yet not across an equivalent waking period. Therefore, sleep may not only modulate affective associations between stimuli but also additionally facilitate their generalization across related contexts.

Nishida and colleagues[53] have demonstrated that sleep, and specifically REM sleep neurophysiology, may underlie such consolidation benefits. Subjects performed 2 study sessions in which they learned emotionally arousing negative and neutral picture stimuli; 1 session was 4 hours prior and 1 was 15 minutes before a recognition memory test. In one group, participants slept (90-minute nap) after the first study session,

whereas in the other group, participants remained awake. Thus, items from the first (4-hour) study sessions transitioned through different brain states in each group before testing, containing sleep in the nap group and no sleep in the no-nap group, yet experienced identical brain-state conditions after the second study session, 15 minutes before testing. No change in memory for emotional (or neutral stimuli) occurred across the offline delay in the no-nap group. However, a significant and selective offline enhancement of emotional memory was observed in the nap group (**Fig. 4**A), the extent of which was correlated with the amount of REM sleep (see **Fig. 4**B), and the speed of entry into REM sleep (latency; not shown in figure). Most striking, spectral analysis of the EEG demonstrated that the magnitude of right-dominant prefrontal theta power during REM sleep (activity in the frequency range of 4.0–7.0 Hz) showed a significant and positive relationship with the amount of emotional memory improvement (see **Fig. 4**C, D).

These findings move beyond demonstrating that affective memories are preferentially enhanced across periods of sleep and indicate that the extent of emotional memory improvement is associated with specific REM sleep characteristics, both quantity and quality (and independent of nocturnal hormonal changes). Corroborating these correlations, it has previously been hypothesized that REM sleep represents a brain-state particularly amenable to emotional memory consolidation, based on its unique biology.[47,54] Neurochemically, levels of limbic and forebrain ACh are markedly elevated during REM sleep,[55,56] reportedly quadruple those seen during NREM and double those measured in quiet waking.[18] Considering the known importance of ACh in the long-term consolidation of emotional learning,[46] this procholinergic REM sleep state may promote the selective memory facilitation of affective memories, similar to that reported using experimental manipulations of ACh.[57] Neurophysiologically, theta oscillations have been proposed as a carrier frequency, allowing disparate brain regions that initially encode information to selectively interact offline, in a coupled relationship. By doing so, REM sleep theta may afford the ability to strengthen distributed aspects of specific memory representations across related but different anatomic networks.[58,59]

Sleep and Emotional Regulation

Relative to the interaction between sleep and affective memory, the effect of sleep loss on basic regulation and perception of emotions has

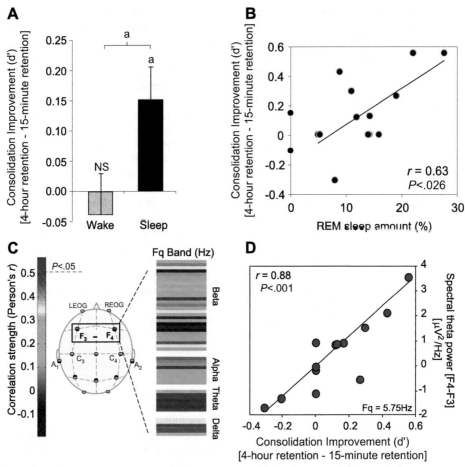

Fig. 4. REM sleep enhancement of negative emotional memories. (*A*) Offline benefit (change in memory recall for 4-hour-old vs 15-minute-old memories) across the day (wake, *gray bar*) or after a 90-minute nap (sleep, *filled bar*). (*B*) Correlation between the amount of offline emotional memory improvement in the nap group (ie, the offline benefit expressed in filled bar of *panel A*), and the amount of REM sleep obtained within the nap. (*C*) Correlation strength (Pearson's *r*-value) between offline benefit for emotional memory in the sleep group (the benefit expressed in filled bar of Fig. A) and the relative right versus left prefrontal spectral-band power (F4–F3) within the delta, alpha, theta, and beta spectral bands, expressed in average 0.5 Hz bin increments. Correlation strength is represented by the color range, demonstrating significant correlations within the theta frequency band (hot colors), and (*D*) exhibiting a maximum significance at the 5.75 Hz bin. [a]*P*<.05; error bars indicate standard error of mean. (*Modified from* Nishida M, Pearsall J, Buckner RL, et al. REM sleep, prefrontal theta, and the consolidation of human emotional memory. Cereb Cortex 2009;19:1158–66; with permission.)

received substantially less research attention. Nevertheless, several studies evaluating subjective as well as objective measures of mood and affect, offer an emerging experimental understanding for the crucial role sleep plays in regulating emotional brain function, complimenting a rich associated clinical literature.

SLEEP LOSS, MOOD STABILITY, AND EMOTIONAL BRAIN (RE)ACTIVITY

Together with impairments of attention and alertness, sleep deprivation is commonly associated with increased subjective reports of irritability and affective volatility.[60] Using a sleep restriction paradigm (5 hours/night), Dinges and colleagues[61] have reported a progressive increase in emotional disturbance across a 1-week period based on questionnaire mood scales. In addition, subjective descriptions in the daily journals of the participants also indicated increasing complaints of emotional difficulties. Zohar and colleagues[62] have investigated the effects of sleep disruption on emotional reactivity to daytime work events in medical residents. Sleep loss was shown to amplify negative emotional consequences of disruptive daytime experiences while blunting the positive benefit associated with rewarding or goal-enhancing activities.

Although these findings help to characterize the behavioral irregularities imposed by sleep loss, evidence for the role of sleep in regulating psychophysiologic reactivity and emotional brain networks is starting to emerge only now. To date, only 2 studies have addressed this interaction. Using functional magnetic resonance imaging (fMRI), Yoo and colleagues[63] examined the effect of 1 night of sleep deprivation on emotional brain reactivity in healthy young adults. During scanning, participants performed an affective stimulus-viewing task involving the presentation of picture slides ranging in a gradient from emotionally neutral to increasingly negative and aversive. Although both groups expressed significant amygdala activation in response to increasingly negative picture stimuli, those in the sleep-deprivation condition showed a remarkable 60% greater magnitude of amygdala reactivity, relative to the control group (**Fig. 5**A, B). In addition to this increased intensity of activation, there was also

a marked increase in the extent of amygdala volume recruited in response to the aversive stimuli in the sleep-deprivation group (see **Fig. 5**B). Relative to the sleep-control group, those who were sleep deprived showed a significant loss of functional connectivity identified between the amygdala and the medial prefrontal cortex, a region known to have strong inhibitory projections to the amygdala (see **Fig. 5**C, D).[64] In contrast, significantly greater connectivity was observed between the amygdala and the autonomic-activating centers of the locus coeruleus in the deprivation group. Therefore, without sleep, an amplified hyperlimbic reaction by the human amygdala was observed in response to negative emotional stimuli, associated with a loss of top-down connectivity with the prefrontal lobe. A similar pattern of anatomic dysfunction has been implicated in several psychiatric mood disorders, which express co-occurring sleep abnormalities[65–67] and directly raises the issue of

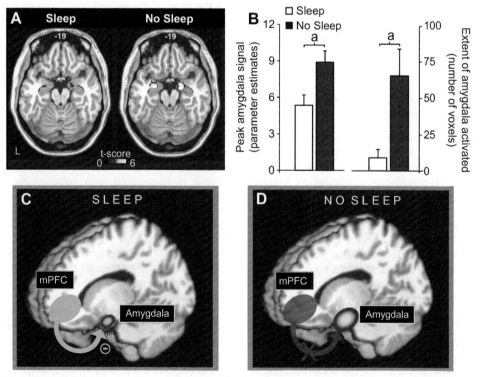

Fig. 5. The effect of sleep deprivation on emotional brain reactivity and functional connectivity. (*A*) Amygdala response to increasingly negative emotional stimuli in the sleep deprivation and sleep-control groups. (*B*) Corresponding differences in intensity and volumetric extent of amygdala activation between the 2 groups (average ± standard error of mean (SEM) of left and right amygdala). (*C*) Depiction of associated changes in functional connectivity between the medial prefrontal cortex (mPFC) and the amygdala. With sleep, the prefrontal lobe was strongly connected to the amygdala, regulating and exerting and inhibitory top-down control. (*D*) Without sleep, however, amygdala-mPFC connectivity was decreased, potentially negating top-down control and resulting in an overactive amygdala. [a]*P*<.01; error bars indicate SEM. (*Modified from* Yoo SS, Gujar N, Hu P, et al. The human emotional brain without sleep—a prefrontal amygdala disconnect. Curr Biol 2007;17:R877; with permission.)

whether sleep loss plays a causal role in the initiation or maintenance of clinical mood disorders.

Complementing these findings, Franzen and colleagues[68] have examined the effect of total sleep deprivation on pupil diameter responses (a measure of autonomic reactivity) during a passive affective picture viewing task containing positive, negative, and neutral stimuli.[68] Relative to a sleep-control group, there was a significantly larger pupillary response to negative pictures compared with positive or neutral stimuli in the deprivation group. Most recently, Gujar and colleagues[69] have compared the change in reactivity to specific types of emotions (fear, anger, happiness, sadness) across a 6 hour daytime waking interval that either did or did not contain a 90-minute nap. Without sleep, reactivity and intensity ratings toward threat-relevant negative emotions (anger and fear) significantly increased with continued time awake. However, an intervening nap blocked (anger) and even reversed (fear) these increases toward aversive stimuli, while conversely enhancing sensitivity toward reward-relevant happy facial expressions. Only those subjects in the nap group who obtained REM sleep displayed this resetting of affective reactivity.

A HEURISTIC MODEL OF SLEEP-DEPENDENT EMOTIONAL PROCESSING

Based on the emerging interaction between sleep and emotion, a synthesis of these findings is provided next, which converge on a functional role for sleep in affective brain modulation. A model of sleep-dependent emotional information processing is described, offering provisional brain-based explanatory insights on the effect of sleep abnormalities in the initiation and maintenance of certain mood disorders and leading to testable predictions for future experimental investigations.

The findings discussed earlier suggest a predisposition for the encoding of negative emotional memories and a hyperlimbic reactivity to negative emotional events under conditions of sleep loss, together with a strengthening of negative memories during subsequent REM sleep, all of which have potential relevance for the understanding of major depression. Thus, at both stages of early memory processing, that is, encoding and consolidation, the architectural sleep abnormalities expressed in major depression may facilitate an adverse prevalence and strengthening of prior negative episodic memories. Yet, there may be an additional consequence of sleep-dependent memory processing, beyond the strengthening of the experience itself, and one that has additional implications for mood disorders – that is, sleeping to forget.

EMOTIONAL MEMORY PROCESSING: A SLEEP TO FORGET AND SLEEP TO REMEMBER HYPOTHESIS

Founded on the emerging interaction between sleep and emotion, the authors outline a model of affective information processing that may offer brain-based explanatory insights regarding the effect of sleep abnormalities, particularly REM sleep, on the initiation or maintenance of mood disturbance.

Although there is abundant evidence to suggest that emotional experiences persist in our autobiographies over time, an equally remarkable but less noted change is a reduction in the affective tone associated with their recall. Affective experiences seem to be encoded and consolidated more robustly than neutral memories because of the autonomic neurochemical reactions elicited at the time of the experience,[46] creating what is commonly termed an emotional memory. However, the later recall of these memories tends not to be associated anywhere near the same magnitude of autonomic (re)activation as that elicited at the moment of experience, suggesting that, over time, the affective "blanket" previously enveloping the memory during learning has been removed, whereas the information contained within that experience (ie, the memory) remains.

For example, neuroimaging studies have shown that the initial exposure and learning of emotional stimuli is associated with substantially greater activation in the amygdala and hippocampus, relative to neutral stimuli.[33,70,71] In 1 of these studies,[33] however, when participants were reexposed to these same stimuli during recognition testing many months later, a change in the profile of activation occurred.[70] Although the same magnitude of differential activity between emotional and neutral items was observed in the hippocampus, this was not true in the amygdala. Instead, the difference in amygdala (re)activity to emotional items compared with neutral items had dissipated over time. This finding may support the idea that the strength of the memory (hippocampus-associated activity) remains at later recollection, yet the associated emotional reactivity to these items (limbic network activity) is reduced over time.

This hypothesis predicts that such decoupling preferentially takes place overnight; such that we sleep to forget the emotional tone, yet sleep to remember the tagged memory of that episode (SFSR model; **Fig. 6**). The model further argues that if this process is not achieved, the magnitude

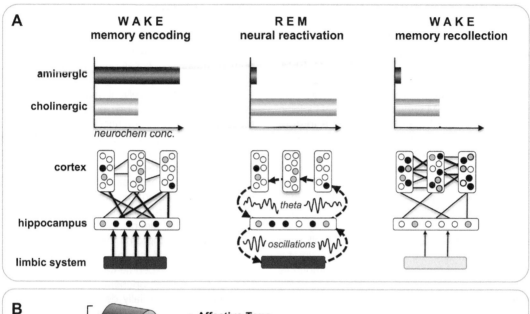

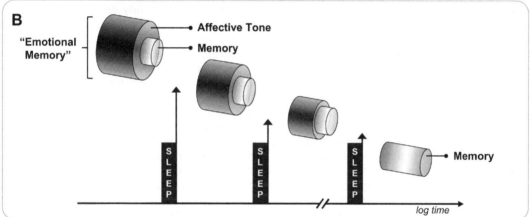

Fig. 6. The sleep to forget and sleep to remember model of emotional memory processing. (*A*) Neural dynamics. Waking formation of an episodic emotional memory involves the coordinated encoding of hippocampal-bound information within cortical modules, facilitated by the extended limbic system, including the amygdala, and modulated by high concentrations of aminergic neurochemistry. During subsequent REM sleep, these same neural structures are reactivated, the coordination of which is made possible by synchronous theta oscillations throughout these networks, supporting the ability to reprocess previously learned emotional experiences. However, this reactivation occurs in a neurochemical milieu devoid of aminergic modulation and dominated by cholinergic neurochemistry. As a consequence, emotional memory reprocessing can achieve, on one hand, a depotentiation of the affective tone initially associated with the events at encoding, while on the other, a simultaneous and progressive neocortical consolidation of the information. The latter process of developing stronger corticocortical connections additionally supports integration into previous acquired autobiographical experiences, further aiding the assimilation of the affective events in the context of past knowledge, the conscious expression of which may contribute to the experience of dreaming. Cross-connectivity between structures is represented by number and thickness of lines. Circles within cortical and hippocampal structures represent information nodes; shade reflects extent of connectivity: strong (*filled*), moderate (*gray*), and weak (*clear*). Fill of limbic system and arrow thickness represent the magnitude of co-activation with and influence on the hippocampus. (*B*) Conceptual outcome. Through multiple iterations of this REM mechanism across the night and/or across multiple nights, the long-term consequence of such sleep-dependent reprocessing would allow for the strengthening and retention of salient information previously tagged as emotional at the time of learning. However, recall no longer maintains an affective, aminergic charge, allowing for postsleep recollection with minimal autonomic reactivity (unlike encoding), thereby preventing a state of chronic anxiety.

of affective charge remaining within autobiographical memory networks would persist, resulting in the potential condition of chronic anxiety or post-traumatic stress disorder (PTSD).

Based on the unique neurobiology of REM, a REM sleep hypothesis of emotional brain processing (see **Fig. 6**A) is proposed. It is suggested that the state of REM provides an optimal biologic theater, within which can be achieved a form of affective "therapy." First, increased activity within limbic and paralimbic structures during REM sleep may first offer the ability for reactivation of previously acquired affective experiences. Second, the neurophysiologic signature of REM sleep involving dominant theta oscillations within subcortical as well as cortical nodes may offer large-scale network cooperation at night, allowing the integration and, as a consequence, greater understanding of recently experienced emotional events in the context of pre-existing neocortically stored semantic memory. Third, these interactions during REM sleep (and perhaps through the conscious process of dreaming) critically and perhaps most importantly take place within a brain that is devoid of aminergic neurochemical concentration,[52] particularly noradrenergic input from the locus coeruleus; the influence of which has been linked to states of high stress and anxiety disorders.[72] Therefore, the neuroanatomical, neurophysiologic, and neurochemical conditions of REM sleep may offer a unique biologic milieu in which to achieve, on one hand, a balanced neural facilitation of the informational core of emotional experiences (the memory), yet may also depotentiate and ultimately ameliorate the autonomic arousing charge originally acquired at the time of learning (the emotion), negating a long-term state of anxiety (see **Fig. 6**).

Specific predictions emerge from this model. First, if this process of seperating emotion from memory was not achieved across the first night after such an experience, the model would predict that a repeat attempt of affective demodulation would occur on the second night, because the strength of the emotional "tag" associated with the memory would remain high. If this process failed a second time, the same events would continue to repeat across ensuing nights. It is just such a cycle of REM-sleep dreaming (nightmares) that represents a diagnostic key feature of PTSD.[73] It may not be coincidental, therefore, that these patients continue to display hyperarousal reactions to associated trauma cues,[74,75] indicating that the process of separating the affective tone from the emotional experience has not been accomplished. The reason why such a REM mechanism may fail in PTSD

remains unknown, although the exceptional magnitude of trauma-induced emotion at the time of learning may be so great that the system is incapable of initiating or completing one or both of these processes, leaving some patients unable to integrate and depotentiate the stored experience. Alternatively, it may be the hyper-arousal status of the brain during REM sleep in these patients,[74–76] potentially lacking sufficient aminergic demodulation, that prevents the processing and separation of emotion from memory. Indeed, this hypothesis has gained support from recent pharmacologic studies in patients with PTSD, demonstrating that nocturnal α-adrenergic blockade using prazosin (ie, reducing adrenergic activity during sleep) both decreases the trauma-dream symptoms and restores the characteristics of REM sleep.[77–79] This model also makes specific experimental predictions on the fate of these 2 components, the memory and the emotion. As partially demonstrated, the first prediction would be that, over time, the veracity of the memory itself would be maintained or improved, and the extent to which these (negative) emotional experiences are strengthened would be proportional to the amount of postexperience REM sleep obtained, as well as how quickly it is achieved (REM latency).

Second, using physiology measures, these same predictions would hold in the inverse direction for the magnitude of emotional reactivity induced at the time of recall. Together with the neuroimaging studies of emotional memory recall over time and psychological studies investigating the role of REM sleep dreaming in mood regulation, a recent fMRI study offers perhaps the strongest preliminary support of this sleep-dependent model of emotional memory processing.[80] Relative to a control group that slept, participants who were deprived of sleep the first night after learning arousing emotion picture slides not only showed reduced recall of the information 72 hours later (the sleep to remember component of the hypothesis) but also showed a lack of reduction in amygdala reactivity when reexposed to these same negative emotional picture slides at recognition testing (**Fig. 7**; the sleep to forget component of the hypothesis). Thus, sleep after learning facilitated improved recollection of these prior emotional experiences, yet this later recollection was conversely associated with a reduction in amygdala reactivity after 3 nights. In contrast, participants who did not sleep the first night after the emotional learning session, despite obtaining 2 full recovery nights of sleep, showed no such depotentiation of subsequent amygdala reactivity.

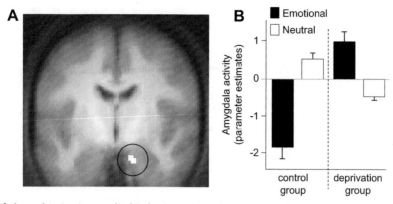

Fig. 7. Effect of sleep deprivation on limbic brain activity during subsequent emotional memory retrieval. (*A*) Higher degree of amygdala reactivity during delayed (72 hours) recollection of previously learned negative emotion picture slides in participants who were sleep deprived the first night after learning, compared with a control group that slept the first night after learning. (*B*) The associated magnetic resonance signal from the amygdala in both groups of subjects, demonstrating a significant reduction in limbic reactivity in those who slept the first night after learning, together with the magnitude of response from the same region to neutral stimulus recollection. (*Modified from* Sterpenich V, Albouy G, Boly M, et al. Sleep-related hippocampo-cortical interplay during emotional memory recollection. PLoS Biol 2007;5:e282; with permission.)

SUMMARY

When viewed as a whole, findings at the cellular, systems, cognitive, and clinical level all point to a crucial role for sleep in the affective modulation of human brain function. Based on the remarkable neurobiology of sleep, and REM sleep in particular, a unique capacity for the overnight modulation of affective networks and previously encountered emotional experiences may be possible, redressing and maintaining the appropriate connectivity and hence the next-day reactivity throughout limbic and associated autonomic systems. However, if the canonical architecture and amount of sleep is disrupted, as commonly occurring in mood disorders, particularly major depression and PTSD, this symbiotic alliance of sleep-dependent emotional brain processing may fail. The predicted consequences of this failure seem to support the development and/or maintenance of several clinical symptoms expressed in mood disorders, whereas the changes in sleep associated with common pharmacologic treatments of these cohorts support a relief of these aberrant overnight processes, all of which lead to experimentally testable hypotheses which can serve to guide future research. Ultimately, the timeless wisdom of mothers alike may never have been more relevant; that is, when troubled "get to bed, you'll feel better in the morning."

REFERENCES

1. Labar KS, Cabeza R. Cognitive neuroscience of emotional memory. Nat Rev Neurosci 2006;7:54.
2. Phelps EA. Emotion and cognition: insights from studies of the human amygdala. Annu Rev Psychol 2006;57:27.
3. Walker MP, Stickgold R. Sleep, memory and plasticity. Annu Rev Psychol 2006;10:139.
4. Rechtschaffen A, Kales A. A manual standardized terminology, techniques and scoring system for sleep stages of human subjects. Bethesda (MD): USA: U.S. Department of Health; 1968.
5. Walker MP. The role of sleep in cognition and emotion. Ann N Y Acad Sci 2009;1156:168–97.
6. Steriade M, Amzica F. Coalescence of sleep rhythms and their chronology in corticothalamic networks. Sleep Res Online 1998;1:1.
7. Armitage R. Sleep and circadian rhythms in mood disorders. Acta Psychiatr Scand Suppl 2007;104.
8. Aston-Jones G, Bloom FE. Activity of norepinephrine-containing locus coeruleus neurons in behaving rats anticipates fluctuations in the sleep-waking cycle. J Neurosci 1981;1:876.
9. Llinas R, Ribary U. Coherent 40-Hz oscillation characterizes dream state in humans. Proc Natl Acad Sci U S A 1993;90:2078.
10. Steriade M, Amzica F, Contreras D. Synchronization of fast (30–40 Hz) spontaneous cortical rhythms during brain activation. J Neurosci 1996; 16:392.
11. Canli T, Zhao Z, Brewer J, et al. Event-related activation in the human amygdala associates with later memory for individual emotional experience. J Neurosci 2000;20:RC99.
12. Saper CB, Chou TC, Scammell TE. The sleep switch: hypothalamic control of sleep and wakefulness. Trends Neurosci 2001;24:726.

13. Hobson JA, McCarley RW, Wyzinski PW. Sleep cycle oscillation: reciprocal discharge by two brainstem neuronal groups. Science 1975;189:55.

14. Lydic R, Baghdoyan HA. Handbook of behavioral state control: cellular and molecular mechanisms. Boca Raton (FL): CRC Press; 1988.

15. Atienza M, Cantero JL. Modulatory effects of emotion and sleep on recollection and familiarity. J Sleep Res 2008;17:285.

16. Shima K, Nakahama H, Yamamoto M. Firing properties of two types of nucleus raphe dorsalis neurons during the sleep-waking cycle and their responses to sensory stimuli. Brain Res 1986; 399:317.

17. Kametani H, Kawamura H. Alterations in acetylcholine release in the rat hippocampus during sleep-wakefulness detected by intracerebral dialysis. Life Sci 1990;47:421.

18. Marrosu F, Portas C, Mascia MS, et al. Microdialysis measurement of cortical and hippocampal acetylcholine release during sleep-wake cycle in freely moving cats. Brain Res 1995;671:329.

19. Nofzinger EA. Functional neuroimaging of sleep. Semin Neurol 2005;25:9.

20. Marshall L, Born J. The contribution of sleep to hippocampus-dependent memory consolidation. Trends Cogn Sci 2007;11:442.

21. Walker MP, Stickgold R. Sleep-dependent learning and memory consolidation. Neuron 2004;44:121.

22. Phelps EA. Human emotion and memory: interactions of the amygdala and hippocampal complex. Curr Opin Neurobiol 2004;14:198.

23. Heuer F, Reisberg D. Vivid memories of emotional events: the accuracy of remembered minutiae. Mem Cognit 1990;18:496–506.

24. Bradley MM, Greenwald MK, Petry MC, et al. Remembering pictures: pleasure and arousal in memory. J Exp Psychol Learn Mem Cogn 1992;18: 379–90.

25. Buchanan TW, Lovallo WR. Enhanced memory for emotional material following stress-level cortisol treatment in humans. Psychoneuroendocrinology 2001;26:307–17.

26. Christianson SA. Emotional stress and eyewitness memory: a critical review. Psycho Bull 1992;112: 284–309.

27. Adolphs R, Cahill L, Schul R, et al. Impaired declarative memory for emotional material following bilateral amygdala damage in humans. Learn Mem 1997;4:291.

28. Cahill L, Prins B, Weber M, et al. Beta-adrenergic activation and memory for emotional events. Nature 1994;371:702.

29. Strange BA, Hurlemann R, Dolan RJ. An emotion-induced retrograde amnesia in humans is amygdala- and beta-adrenergic-dependent. Proc Natl Acad Sci U S A 2003;100:13626.

30. Amzica F, Steriade M. Short- and long-range neuronal synchronization of the slow (<1 Hz) cortical oscillation. J Neurophysiol 1995;73:20.

31. Cahill L, Haier RJ, Fallon J, et al. Amygdala activity at encoding correlated with long-term, free recall of emotional information. Proc Natl Acad Sci U S A 1996;93:8016.

32. Conway MA, Anderson SJ, Larsen SF, et al. The formation of flashbulb memories. Mem Cognit 1994; 22:326.

33. Dolcos F, LaBar KS, Cabeza R. Interaction between the amygdala and the medial temporal lobe memory system predicts better memory for emotional events. Neuron 2004;42:855.

34. Hamann SB, Ely TD, Grafton ST, et al. Amygdala activity related to enhanced memory for pleasant and aversive stimuli. Nat Neurosci 1999;2:289.

35. Kensinger EA, Corkin S. Two routes to emotional memory: distinct neural processes for valence and arousal. Proc Natl Acad Sci U S A 2004;101:3310.

36. Sharot T, Phelps EA. How arousal modulates memory: disentangling the effects of attention and retention. Cogn Affect Behav Neurosci 2004; 4:294.

37. Harrison Y, Horne JA. Sleep loss and temporal memory. Q J Exp Psychol 2000;53:271.

38. Morris GO, Williams HL, Lubin A. Misperception and disorientation during sleep. Arch Gen Psychiatry 1960;2:247.

39. Yoo SS, Hu PT, Gujar N, et al. A deficit in the ability to form new human memories without sleep. Nat Neurosci 2007;10:385.

40. Buzsaki G. Theta oscillations in the hippocampus. Neuron 2002;33:325.

41. Kleinsmith LJ, Kaplan S. Paired-associate learning as a function of arousal and interpolated interval. J Exp Psychol 1963;65:190.

42. LaBar KS, Phelps EA. Arousal-mediated memory consolidation: role of the medial temporal lobe in humans. Psychol Sci 1998;9:490.

43. Levonian E. Retention over time in relation to arousal during learning: an explanation of discrepant results. Acta Psychol (Amst) 1972;36:290.

44. Walker EL, Tarte RD. Memory storage as a function of arousal and time with homogeneous and heterogeneous lists. J Verb Learn Verb Behav 1963;2:113.

45. Cahill L, Babinsky R, Markowitsch HJ, et al. The amygdala and emotional memory. Nature 1995; 377:295.

46. McGaugh JL. The amygdala modulates the consolidation of memories of emotionally arousing experiences. Annu Rev Neurosci 2004;27:1.

47. Hu P, Stylos-Allen M, Walker MP. Sleep facilitates consolidation of emotionally arousing declarative memory. Psychol Sci 2006;17:891.

48. Wagner U, Gais S, Born J. Emotional memory formation is enhanced across sleep intervals with high

amounts of rapid eye movement sleep. Learn Mem 2001;8:112.

49. Wagner U, Hallschmid M, Rasch B, et al. Brief sleep after learning keeps emotional memories alive for years. Biol Psychiatry 2006;60:788.

50. Wagner U, Kashyap N, Diekelmann S, et al. The impact of post-learning sleep vs. wakefulness on recognition memory for faces with different facial expressions. Neurobiol Learn Mem 2007;87:679.

51. Payne JD, Stickgold R, Swanberg K, et al. Sleep preferentially enhances memory for emotional components of scenes. Psychol Sci 2008;19:781.

52. Pace-Schott EF, Hobson JA. The neurobiology of sleep: genetics, cellular physiology and subcortical networks. Nat Rev Neurosci 2002;3:591.

53. Nishida M, Pearsall J, Buckner RL, et al. REM sleep, prefrontal theta, and the consolidation of human emotional memory. Cereb Cortex 2009;19:1158.

54. Pare D, Collins DR, Pelletier JG. Amygdala oscillations and the consolidation of emotional memories. Trends Cogn Sci 2002;6:306.

55. Vazquez J, Baghdoyan HA. Basal forebrain acetylcholine release during REM sleep is significantly greater than during waking. Am J Physiol Regul Integr Comp Physiol 2001;280:R598.

56. Wagner U, Fischer S, Born J. Changes in emotional responses to aversive pictures across periods rich in slow-wave sleep versus rapid eye movement sleep. Psychosom Med 2002;64:627.

57. Power AE. Muscarinic cholinergic contribution to memory consolidation: with attention to involvement of the basolateral amygdala. Curr Med Chem 2004; 11:987.

58. Cahill L. Neurobiological mechanisms of emotionally influenced, long-term memory. Prog Brain Res 2000; 126:29.

59. Jones MW, Wilson MA. Theta rhythms coordinate hippocampal-prefrontal interactions in a spatial memory task. PLoS Biol 2005;3:e402.

60. Horne JA. Sleep function, with particular reference to sleep deprivation. Ann Clin Res 1985;17:199.

61. Dinges DF, Pack F, Williams K, et al. Cumulative sleepiness, mood disturbance, and psychomotor vigilance performance decrements during a week of sleep restricted to 4–5 hours per night. Sleep 1997;20:267.

62. Zohar D, Tzischinsky O, Epstein R, et al. The effects of sleep loss on medical residents' emotional reactions to work events: a cognitive energy model. Sleep 2005;28:47.

63. Yoo SS, Gujar N, Hu P, et al. The human emotional brain without sleep—a prefrontal amygdala disconnect. Curr Biol 2007;17:R877.

64. Sotres-Bayon F, Bush DE, LeDoux JE. Emotional perseveration: an update on prefrontal-amygdala interactions in fear extinction. Learn Mem 2004; 11:525.

65. Davidson RJ. Anxiety and affective style: role of prefrontal cortex and amygdala. Biol Psychiatry 2002;51:68.

66. Davidson RJ, Pizzagalli D, Nitschke JB, et al. Depression: perspectives from affective neuroscience. Annu Rev Psychol 2002;53:545.

67. New AS, Hazlett EA, Buchsbaum MS, et al. Amygdala-prefrontal disconnection in borderline personality disorder. Neuropsychopharmacology 2007;32:1629.

68. Franzen PL, Buysse DJ, Dahl RE, et al. Sleep deprivation alters pupillary reactivity to emotional stimuli in healthy young adults. Biological Psychology 2009;80:300–5.

69. Gujar N, McDonald SA, Nishida M, et al. A role for REM sleep in recalibrating the sensitivity of the human brain to specific emotions. Cereb Cortex 2011;21(1):115.

70. Dolcos F, LaBar KS, Cabeza R. Remembering one year later: role of the amygdala and the medial temporal lobe memory system in retrieving emotional memories. Proc Natl Acad Sci U S A 2005;102:2626.

71. Kilpatrick L, Cahill L. Amygdala modulation of parahippocampal and frontal regions during emotionally influenced memory storage. Neuroimage 2003;20: 2091.

72. Sullivan GM, Coplan JD, Kent JM, et al. The noradrenergic system in pathological anxiety: a focus on panic with relevance to generalized anxiety and phobias. Biol Psychiatry 1999;46:1205.

73. Lavie P. Sleep disturbances in the wake of traumatic events. N Engl J Med 2001;345:1825.

74. Harvey AG, Jones C, Schmidt DA. Sleep and posttraumatic stress disorder: a review. Clin Psychol Rev 2003;23:377.

75. Pole N. The psychophysiology of posttraumatic stress disorder: a meta-analysis. Psychol Bull 2007;133:725.

76. Strawn JR, Geracioti TD Jr. Noradrenergic dysfunction and the psychopharmacology of posttraumatic stress disorder. Depress Anxiety 2008; 25:260.

77. Raskind MA, Peskind ER, Hoff DJ, et al. A parallel group placebo controlled study of prazosin for trauma nightmares and sleep disturbance in combat veterans with post-traumatic stress disorder. Biol Psychiatry 2007;61:928.

78. Taylor FB, Martin P, Thompson C, et al. Prazosin effects on objective sleep measures and clinical symptoms in civilian trauma posttraumatic stress disorder: a placebo-controlled study. Biol Psychiatry 2008;63:629.

79. Tsuno N, Besset A, Ritchie K. Sleep and depression. J Clin Psychiatry 2005;66:1254.

80. Sterpenich V, Albouy G, Boly M, et al. Sleep-related hippocampo-cortical interplay during emotional memory recollection. PLoS Biol 2007;5:e282.

Learning, Memory, and Sleep in Children

Rebecca L. Gomez, MA, PhD*,
Katharine C. Newman-Smith, BA, Jennifer H. Breslin, MA,
Richard R. Bootzin, MS, PhD

KEYWORDS

• Infants • Children • Adolescents • Learning • Sleep
• Memory • Cognitive outcomes • School achievement

Are we getting enough sleep to learn and function optimally? Sleep loss is endemic in our population, with many adults and children receiving less sleep than needed.[1–3] What are the effects of variations in sleep on childhood learning? Despite a burgeoning literature on sleep and learning in adults[4–6] there is little known about the direct effects of sleep on child learning. There is indirect evidence from developmental work in animals and from correlational work investigating the relationship between children's sleep-wake state organization and their performance on cognitive outcomes, with the literature on long-term disordered sleep also contributing to the understanding of the effects of sleep on childhood learning. More direct evidence comes from a small body of experimental work on restricted sleep in children.[7] Finally, a very small number of studies have begun to investigate the direct effects of sleep on learning by comparing learning after periods of sleep versus wake.[2] Although one might expect continuity in the effects of sleep on learning in children compared with adults, the experimental evidence paints an intriguing, picture, one that is explored in this article along with a review of correlational work investigating the effect of sleep variables on cognitive outcomes in children and experimental work investigating the effects of sleep restriction on learning. The authors begin by providing a brief outline of the development of sleep in children.

DEVELOPMENT OF SLEEP
Gestational Sleep

Sleep plays an essential role in the development and plasticity of the brain.[8] Crucial neurologic growth and development of the primary sensory systems occur both prenatally and postnatally. For typical development, both genetic factors and early experience are highly influential during these critical periods to establish and refine the basic connections.[9,10] Prenatal diagnostics have shown that as the fetus develops in the womb, so does sleep.[11] This development largely parallels the maturation of the fetus' cortex and central nervous system (CNS).[10,12] A cyclic physiologic rhythm oscillating between active and restful states can be identified in the second trimester. Using real-time ultrasonography, these distinct states can be detected by physical movements of the fetus, specifically of the limb and eye.[11,12] Cyclic patterns present in the basic activity-rest cycles are thought to be manifestations of the CNS ultradian rhythm. This ontogeny of sleep continues to develop systematically from the ultradian rhythm during early gestation to characterizable states of active sleep and quiet sleep.[11,13] Around the 25th week of gestation, these sleep states are observable in cycles ranging from 40 to 60 minutes. At 27 to 28 weeks' gestation, the electric patterns of the states are more distinctive, becoming a fully formed sleep cycle at 35 weeks' gestation.[12]

Funding: This work was supported by NSF grant BCS-0743988 to R.L.G. and funding from the Down Syndrome Research and Treatment Foundation supporting J.H.B.
Psychology Department, The University of Arizona, PO Box 210068, Tucson, AZ 85721-0068, USA
* Corresponding author.
E-mail address: rgomez@u.arizona.edu

Sleep Med Clin 6 (2011) 45–57
doi:10.1016/j.jsmc.2010.12.002
1556-407X/11/$ – see front matter © 2011 Elsevier Inc. All rights reserved.

Neonatal and Infant Sleep: Ages 0 to 12 Months

After a full-term birth, occurring between 38 and 42 weeks' gestation, there is rapid development of the neonate's CNS, but until around 6 months of age, the neonatal cortex is unable to sustain the waves that have higher frequency and amplitude that are present in later life sleep. At this stage of development rapid eye movement (REM) and non-REM (NREM) are not yet sufficiently organized identifiable states. Sleep is thus defined in these early months using a combination of electroencephalogram (EEG), respiration, heart rate, and behavioral data.[14]

Using such scoring, there are 3 distinct states of sleep at birth and in the immediate neonatal period, including active, quiet, and indeterminate states. Active sleep is defined electrophysiologically as constant activity throughout the neocortex. Active sleep that precedes quiet sleep is characterized by high-amplitude activity (up to 70 μV), whereas active sleep that follows a period of quiet sleep shows lower-amplitude waves (20–50 μV).[15,16] At this time, cortical activation is not distinguishable between active sleep and wake states, with both states showing similar high-frequency high-amplitude waves.[12] Quiet sleep exhibits a background pattern of noise with alternating bursts of theta and delta waves, with amplitudes up to 200 μV. Periods of quick alpha and beta activity are intermingled in this theta and delta activity, with amplitudes falling between 50 and 70 μV.[14,16] During quiet sleep, these oscillating amplitudes can synchronize in both hemispheres. In these early months, this pattern of sleep is known as trace alternant, after its characteristic changes from high- to low-amplitude activity over the entire neocortex. Trace alternant is also known as discontinuous sleep because of its patterned bursts of initial moderate- to high-voltage activity followed by low-voltage activity.[12,16] The final sleep state is indeterminate, encompassing many of the transitions between identifiable active and quiet sleep and characterized by disorganized EEG signals.[16]

Neonates sleep in polyphasic cycles, sleeping between 12 and 17 hours a day, typically for short periods, from 3 to 4 hours, marked by frequent arousals. Transition to sleep from the waking state is accomplished through an initial short period of active sleep. As the infant matures, this initial period of active sleep disappears and forms into the transition typical of adults, through NREM1. After this initial short period of active sleep, the infant enters the typical alternating cyclic oscillations of active/quiet sleep, similar to that of adults,

with the infant sleep cycles typically lasting 50 minutes as compared with the adult cycles of 90 minutes.[12,16] As neonates progress into infancy, their polyphasic sleep begins to normalize, with their sleep architecture becoming more durable and adultlike. As neonates age, the infantile sleep pattern becomes diurnal, and at the age of about 6 months, characterizable REM and NREM sleep states have developed. This change may be caused by the maturation of the infant cortex, which is now able to sustain the high-amplitude waves exhibited in delta sleep.[17] The trace alternant pattern also disappears by 47 weeks postterm, having developed into the known NREM sleep state, with constant fluid delta waves.[12]

The emergence of sleep spindles and K complexes marks the transition from neonatal to infantile sleep. At 8 to 11 weeks postterm, typically developing infants display bursts of activity during NREM2 quiet sleep of 11 to 15 Hz. In the first year of life, the spindle activity becomes identifiable in the sleep state NREM2, showing increased synchrony; the bursts of spindle activity show increases in bilateral synchrony and symmetry as the infant develops, up to 70% at 12 months.[12,14,18,19] Until about 24 months, there is not consistent synchronous spindle activity across the hemispheres.[12] In addition, between the ages of 5 and 6 months, K complexes appear during NREM2. K complexes are brain waves that present as an initial sharp negative high-voltage wave followed by a positive wave.[18] These waves are the classic markers of the transition from neonatal to infant sleep.

Early and Middle Childhood: Ages 1 to 12 Years

During early and middle childhood, sleep and wakeful patterns become more consistent and durable, similar to those of adults. During early childhood, that is, ages 1 to 5 years, children continue to need a modified polyphasic sleep cycle composed of multiple naps during the day and an extended period of sleep at night. In this prepubertal age group, there is a steady decline in the percentage of REM sleep in total sleep time, from around 25% at 12 months of age to 18.5% by 12 years of age.[20] NREM sleep increases slightly during early childhood, and then, it too has a slight gradual decline during this age range.[20] Around the age of 5 years, the polyphasic cycle has ended, and nocturnal sleep is typically between 10 to 12 hours, with at most one nap during the day.[21] Between the ages of 4.5 and 7 years, sleep is marked by latent REM. Before this age, children typically ascend into the first period of REM after accomplishing NREM1 to 3, yet during these ages REM sleep is entered only after 3 to 4 cycles of NREM sleep. This latent REM is thought to be driven by a NREM drive, which may result from increases in physical activity.[20] As the child ages, this latent REM pattern disappears and sleep returns to a more typical adultlike pattern, with REM appearing 50 to 70 minutes after sleep begins.

Aside from decline in REM sleep, middle childhood sleep is characterized by few architectural changes. Rather, modifications occur in sleep behaviors because of changing life factors. Between the ages of 7 and 12 years, day napping becomes nonexistent and total nocturnal sleep time decreases to between 8.5 to 10.5 hours.[21,22] While wake time remains constant across this age range, bedtimes are delayed consistently by age.[23] During this time, socioenvironmental factors expand and intensify, including increased social activities and access to television, video games, and computers, leading to large alterations in sleep behavior by adolescence.[23]

Adolescence: Ages 12 to 18 Years

Increased psychosocial pressures and biologic changes mark the period between childhood and adulthood, all leading to a temporary transformation of the sleep-wake cycle. Sleep homeostasis, the regulation of the sleep-wake cycle, is affected by the biologic sexual maturation of puberty and the attenuation of sleep opportunity caused by enhanced amounts of schoolwork, earlier school start times, intensified extracurricular activities, and social obligations.[22,24–26] Seen in the adolescent, sleep preference is a tendency toward phase delay, composed of later bedtime and wake times. However, because of the aforementioned circumstances, the typical adolescent is chronically sleep deprived.[22,25] Sexual maturation is thought to play a key role in this alteration of the sleep-wake patterns.[22] During this time, sleep is regulated by the interaction of a 2-process model, the dependent Process S, which involves the homeostatic sleep pressure, and the independent Process C, involving the biologic mechanisms affecting sleep. Process S is a feedback sleep drive system. As wake time mounts, our sleep drive builds, resetting only with the onset and accomplishment of sleep. Process C is the biologic mechanism of the circadian rhythm. This oscillating biologic rhythm of active and restful states synchronizes to our environmental schedules and constraints, including wake and rest times. The biologic mechanisms involved in Process C include the superchiasmatic nuclei or nucleus, neurotransmitter and hormone secretion, and alterations in body temperature.[27,28] In combination, the sleep homeostasis and circadian processes interact to modify and regulate our sleep-wake cycle, which in the adolescent involves increased total wake time, increased daily sleepiness, and later bedtimes,[22–26] all being changes with implications for memory and learning.

The aforementioned developmental changes in sleep raise several questions for the role of sleep in childhood learning. For instance, given the findings in the adult literature showing that learning diminishes during time awake, we might ask whether immediate sleep is critical during polyphasic periods of sleep when children are still napping frequently. We might also ask whether there is a critical period for the effects of sleep on learning such that early deficits in sleep have greater effect than later deficits. A final question is whether sleep affects learning similarly in children and adults. These and other questions are addressed in the following sections. The authors now focus on correlational research investigating the relationship between sleep and learning.

CORRELATIONAL RELATIONSHIPS BETWEEN SLEEP AND LEARNING

The vast literature using sleep measures to predict cognitive outcomes suggests an important role for sleep in learning in childhood, with fragmented and reduced sleep associated with deficits in cognitive abilities, IQ, and grades at all developmental ages.[18,29,30]

Infants

The Bayley Mental Development Inventory (MDI) has been used widely to assess cognitive development between birth and 42 months. Although limited in its ability to predict future cognitive outcomes,[31] the MDI has been useful as a measure of cognitive development in infancy and toddlerhood and has been particularly instrumental in studies correlating sleep measures with an index of cognitive development. Evidence that more-regulated less-fragmented sleep is associated with more-advanced cognitive development comes from several sources. In data obtained from full night videos of premature infants at 1, 2, 5, 6, 9, and 12 months, the developmental rate of the holding time index, a measure of the length of early-nocturnal quiet sleep periods, was correlated with higher MDI scores at 6 months of age. Furthermore, longer sustained sleep periods, reflecting consistency across development in the ability to sustain long sleep, was associated with higher MDI scores at 1 year.[17] Both measures are thought to capture maturation of sleep. Although sleep cyclicity length at preterm (measured at 36 weeks) was negatively correlated with the 6-month MDI scores, sleep cyclicity at 6 months was positively correlated, with a similar pattern found for amounts of active sleep.[32] One interpretation of the negative correlations in the preterm period is that longer sleep cyclicity and greater amounts of active sleep are reactions to the stress associated with the many medical interventions required for preterm infants.[32] In a study using actigraphy to investigate sleep in older infants, high sleep efficiency in a group of 50 healthy full-term infants was positively correlated with the MDI scores at 10 months, whereas motor activity during sleep and greater numbers of night arousals were negatively correlated.[33] Finally, infants with better circadian sleep regulation at 7 and 19 months (obtained from parental report and reflected in the proportion of variance in the sleep-wake cycle accounted for by circadian rhythm) had higher MDI scores at 24 months and higher receptive and expressive language skill at 36 months. The rate of growth in circadian sleep regulation was also positively correlated with the MDI score at 24 months.[34]

A more complicated picture emerges when measures of sleep are obtained immediately after birth or during a period of greater compromise in development. Longer mean sleep periods, longest sustained sleep periods, shorter sleep-wake transitions, and more arousals in quiet sleep obtained from 36 full-term infants on day 1 were associated with lower MDI scores at 6 months, whereas there were no significant correlations based on day 2 sleep data.[35] Although the negative correlations for the first 2 measures are contrary to what might be expected, they may reflect a reaction to the stress of birth, with stronger reactions being a greater predictor of developmental vulnerability as reflected in lower MDI scores. That stress might be associated with longer quiet sleep is supported by studies in newborns, showing that excessive stimulation or pain is associated with longer durations of quiet sleep,[36] and also in a study measuring sleep in 16 premature and 16 full-term infants at 40 weeks' conceptional age (CA), in which less-developed active sleep (as reflected in fewer REMs per minute) and shorter sleep-wake transitions were also associated with lower MDI scores at 12 and 24 months.[37] Similarly, when the proportion of REM in active sleep was assessed in 81 premature infants between 32 and 36 weeks' CA, low REM activity predicted lower MDI scores at 6 months.[38] Using actigraphy in 34 premature infants, lower total nighttime sleep and higher mean nighttime activity at 36 weeks'

CA (but not at 32 weeks) were associated with higher MDI scores at 6 months, a finding that would seem to contradict those described earlier.[39] The investigators argued that to the extent that total night activity reflects active sleep, such sleep may facilitate growth and maturation by stimulating the nervous system.[40] This argument is corroborated in a study reporting higher incidences of night arousals associated with higher MDI scores.[37] However, higher levels of snoring-related arousals in the absence of apnea or hypopnea were associated with lower MDI scores in 35 infants aged 8 months, with the frequency of arousals during snoring related to the prevalence of smoke in the household.[41]

The effects of sleep variation in infancy can also be traced through later childhood. In one study with 53 premature infants, the percentage of trace alternate EEGs occurring in quiet sleep at 40 weeks' CA correlated with Gesell developmental scores at 4, 9, and 24 months of age; Stanford-Binet Test scores at 5 years of age; and scores on the Wechsler Intelligence Scale for Children (WISC) as far out as 8 years of age.[42] Although the Gesell developmental test provides a composite assessment of development, including social, emotional, physical, and adaptive factors, it also incorporates cognitive development. In a study obtaining weekly sleep observations of 51 preterm infants, more rapid development of active sleep, involving greater proportions of REM in active sleep and more rapidly decreasing proportions of active to quiet sleep, was associated with higher Stanford-Binet IQ scores and more advanced expressive language skill at the age of 3 years.[43] In addition, less time spent in active sleep in premature infants at 40 weeks was related to greater learning problems and greater distractability at the age of 8 years.[44] Finally, in a study investigating REM in 2 groups of 14 to 15 full-term infants at 2 to 5 weeks and during the first 2 hours of nighttime sleep at 3, 6, and 9 months, higher rates of REM storms at 6 months were associated with lower Bayley MDI scores at 12 months. REM storms, bursts of REMs in active sleep with very high amplitude, are thought to reflect immature regulation in CNS pathways, with a reduction of REM storms reflecting CNS maturation.[45]

Although the findings converge on the idea that poor sleep in infancy is associated with poorer cognitive development, there are several discrepancies in the findings, resulting perhaps from variations in methodology across studies or from variations in the ages tested. In some cases, operational measures are far from settled, as with determining the defining characteristics of waking episodes.[33,46] In other cases, differences in how researchers score infant sleep or whether they obtain their measures through actigraphy, EEG, or pressure-sensitive mattresses may contribute to variations in the results. Finally, findings showing that predictability can vary across intervals as short as 2 days suggest that fine gradations in when sleep is measured may affect the resulting correlations.[35]

Children and Adolescents

Studies have also investigated the relationship of sleep variables to cognitive and academic measures in childhood and adolescence. Short sleep duration in children aged 2.5 to 6 years (obtained via parental report) has been found to be related to lower receptive vocabulary as measured by the Peabody Picture Vocabulary Test-Revised (PPVT-R) at 5 years and with lower nonverbal intellectual skills as measured on the block design subtest of the WISC-III at 6 years.[47] Children who slept 1 to 1.5 hours less a night over periods of 2 to 6 years (8.5–9.0 hours a night instead of 10 or 11 hours) were thrice as likely to have lower scores on the PPVT-R, suggesting that shorter sleep may impede new word learning. Finally, children who were initially short sleepers (7.5 hours) but recovered normal sleep duration by 3 years were also 2.5 times more likely to have lower scores on the WISC, reflecting an extended effect of shorter sleep in early childhood. In another study using the WISC and reaction time tests with 166 third graders, African American and European American children performed similarly when sleep quality (assessed by actigraphy) was high, but when sleep quality was poor and socioeconomic status (SES) was controlled, the African American children performed more poorly.[48] A similar finding was reported for academic functioning as measured by Stanford-Binet scores with the same sample of children—when the sleep quality was high, children with high and low SES performed similarly, but when the sleep quality was low, children with lower SES performed more poorly on the cognitive tests.[49] However, not all findings are consistent with the picture that less sleep during childhood leads to poorer cognitive performance. A recent study of 60 children aged 7 to 11 years reported that those with higher full-scale WISC intelligence scores had less total sleep on weekends as reported by their parents.[50] Because only 1 child had to wake up for weekend activities, weekend sleep for the rest of the sample may be a more accurate estimate of their underlying sleep pattern than sleep during the week. One possible explanation of the

apparent contradiction with other studies showing that more sleep correlates with better cognitive performance is that more weekend sleep may reflect the development of a delayed sleep phase pattern[51] caused by less-than-adequate sleep during the week.

Other studies have focused on the relationship of sleep to more targeted measures of cognitive functions. In a study with 135 second, fourth, and fifth graders, sleep fragmentation, reflected in more night awakenings and lower sleep efficiency using actigraphy, was related to poorer executive functioning, measured in higher false alarms in a continuous performance task (CPT), a measure of attention and executive function requiring children to respond to a picture of a particular animal but not to pictures of other animals, as well as a symbol digit substitution test, in which children typed a digit paired with a particular symbol in different ordered lists of pairs. Higher correlations in the second graders suggested that younger children might be more vulnerable to sleep disruption than older children.[52] Greater sleep efficiency and shorter sleep latency, as measured by actigraphy, were also related to working memory performance in 60 children aged 6 to 13 years, with more errors associated with lower sleep efficiency and longer latency in an auditory n-back task requiring children to respond to particular spatial locations of an auditory signal.[53] Regarding grades, the incidence of poor school achievement in 1000 elementary-aged school children was higher in children who were poor sleepers as measured by parental report.[54] This outcome was corroborated in a positive correlation between self-reported amount of nighttime sleep and grades in 2259 sixth, seventh, and eighth graders.[55,56]

In later adolescence, 12th graders who did not catch up on lost sleep on the weekends (measured by self-report) had poorer grades than those who caught up on sleep.[57] For students aged 13 to 19 years receiving grades of C and lower, the self-reported sleep time on school nights was 17 to 33 minutes less and the bedtime was 10 to 50 minutes later than students receiving grades A and B.[3] Students with higher grades also went to sleep earlier on weekend nights by as much as half an hour. Related studies report similar findings, with lower school achievement associated with later bedtimes[58] and less habitual sleep[58,59] and higher grade point averages associated with later school rise times, earlier weekend rise times, shorter sleep latency, less fragmented sleep, and fewer daytime naps,[60] however, not all studies find a significant correlation with earlier school start times and poorer academic performance.[61]

Excessive sleepiness has also been associated with lower grades. Students (11–15 years) who slept less had higher levels of daytime sleepiness, which in turn related to poorer school achievement.[62] Excessive sleepiness, assessed on the Epworth Sleepiness Scale, was also associated with poorer final examination grades in 11th graders.[63]

Disordered Childhood Sleep

Finally, the literature on disordered sleep due to snoring (apart from hypoxia) reveals effects on grades,[64] cognitive tests, such as the Wilkinson Addition Test,[65] and attention, memory, and intelligence measures[66] in 5- to 10-year-old children, with improvements in cognitive performance resulting after treatment of snoring.[67] A more fine-grained assessment tested children (6–17 years) with behavioral sleep problems (BSPs), children who snored, children with both these ailments, and children with neither ailment who served as controls. Snoring was associated with a lower IQ and poorer selective attention but not lower memory, whereas BSP was associated with reduced nonverbal memory.[68]

Studies on children with obstructive sleep apnea (OSA) have also been revealing, with children with OSA scoring significantly lower than children without OSA symptoms on tests of attention, executive function, memory, and general intellectual ability.[66,68,69] Mild OSA was associated with impairments in sustained attention and vigilance on the CPT. Associations between OSA and deficits on Developmental NEuroloPSYcological Assessment (NEPSY) subtests of executive function, including the auditory CPT, Tower of London task, and the visual attention, and verbal fluency subtests have also been reported.[70,71] Children with OSA symptoms have been shown to score lower than controls on memory tests, including the Wide Range Assessment of Memory and Learning (WRAML) screening index,[66] the Luria verbal learning task, and the Rey-Osterrieth Complex Figure test.[72] Finally, several recent studies have reported full-scale IQ deficits among children with OSA symptoms relative to controls[71,73–75] (but see[76,77]) and lower school performance.[78–80]

In summary, although the general picture resulting from the literature suggests a relationship between sleep and later cognitive functioning spanning infancy through adolescence, the picture is not always straightforward, with some findings failing to replicate or reflecting conflicting results. Furthermore, with correlational approaches, it is impossible to know whether relationships between

sleep and cognition reflect overall maturation, whether sleep is truly implicated in cognitive outcomes, or whether some other unknown variable is at play.[18] Thus, more direct manipulations of the effects of sleep on memory and learning are needed, such as those involving sleep restriction and/or enhancement.

THE EFFECTS OF SLEEP RESTRICTION ON CHILDHOOD LEARNING

The effect of sleep on learning can be directly investigated by restricting sleep before testing.[7] In a complementary pair of studies, 11- to 14-year-old children were allowed only 4 hours of sleep[81] or were deprived of sleep for a full night.[82] Compromised functioning was observed after a full night of sleep deprivation only, with participants making fewer attempts of an addition task requiring them to add sets of 5 two-digit numbers and poorer memory recall from a list of 25 briefly exposed words. A study in a similar vein also failed to observe differences in response inhibition and sustained attention in a sleep-optimized group of 8- and 15-year old children compared with a group with only 4 hours of sleep,[83] raising the possibility that reduced sleep may specifically affect higher levels of cognition (vs the lower levels manifested in the response-inhibition task and the sustained-attention task used).[84] Children (7–14 years) with 5 hours of sleep performed the same as controls on low-level psychomotor tasks and on a simple memory task but performed worse on the Wisconsin Card Sorting Task, a task of executive control in which participants sort pictures according to dimensions such as color or size.[84] Restricted sleep also interfered with creative thinking as measured in the fluency with which participants generated ideas using words and their flexibility generating different kinds of ideas, different strategies, and switching between them.[84] The finding that mild sleep deprivation does not interfere with low-level cognitive functioning was further replicated in a study with 10-year-old girls who learned a list of 15 words, were exposed to a list of interference items, and then recalled the first list immediately and after 10 or 5 hours of sleep (control and sleep restriction conditions, respectively).[85] This pattern of differences between the control and sleep-restricted groups for high-level but not for low-level cognitive tasks is consistent with those in the adult literature, showing that executive control is particularly vulnerable to sleep deprivation.[86–89]

In a study investigating modest changes in sleep and using teacher ratings of academic functioning, school-aged children (6–12 years) were tested over a period of 3 weeks in which baseline measures of sleep were obtained in week 1, whereas in weeks 2 and 3 the children participated in counterbalanced within-subject manipulations of extended (10 hours sleep) and restricted sleep (8 hours for younger children and 6.5 hours for older children).[90] At the end of each week, children were assessed by their teachers on various measures of their work including quality, percentage completed, how quickly they learned, their retention, and the care with which they executed their work. When sleep was restricted, children were judged by their teachers to learn and process information more slowly, to be less attentive, and to be more forgetful than during their baseline and extended sleep weeks.

In another study of mild sleep restriction, a group of children aged 10 years whose sleep was restricted by 30 minutes or more on 3 successive nights was compared with a group whose sleep was extended by 30 minutes or more.[91] Children who extended their sleep improved their performance significantly compared with baseline on a forward digit-span task (involving working memory) and on CPT (reflecting visual attention and response inhibition) compared with children in the sleep-restricted group suggesting that sleep extension may benefit low- and high-level cognitive tasks similarly. The reaction time performance of the children who extended their sleep was also preserved compared with the sleep-restricted group. Finally, 19 high-school students who extended their sleep by at least 60 minutes on 3 consecutive nights showed reduced daytime sleepiness, improved backward digit span, and improved performance on the Trail-making Test Part B compared with controls who did not extend their sleep.[92]

In summary, partial sleep restriction seems to have similar effects in children and adults, with a greater effect on measures of higher-level prefrontal cognitive functioning than on lower-level functioning. Furthermore, rather small reductions in sleep can affect academic performance and cognitive functioning, whereas extensions in sleep can result in improvements.

DIRECT COMPARISONS OF MEMORY CONSOLIDATION DURING WAKE AND SLEEP

An approach that has been used productively to assess the effects of sleep on learning with adults is to expose them to a learning task before a period of normal wake time or before sleep, with both groups tested after an equal delay. Although continuities in certain forms of child and adult learning might suggest that children would be affected similarly by sleep after learning,[93–97] in fact they are not. Children seem to be affected differently on a measure of procedural (skill-based) learning as compared with declarative (or fact based) learning, as is described in the following section.

In a study investigating the effects of sleep on procedural learning, children (7–11 years) and adults performed a sequential reaction time (SRT) task, a motor learning task requiring them to type a series of keys corresponding to the location of a cursor on the screen.[98] The cursor moved among 6 locations where the 2 preceding locations in sequence predicted 1 of 2 successors, each 50% of the time. Children were tested on their reaction times to respond to legal transitions versus illegal ones that had never followed the 2 preceding locations. Children and adults learned in the evening and were tested approximately 11.5 hours (children) or 10.5 hours later (adults) after sleep. The same subjects participated in a wake condition, learning in the morning and testing at night (with equivalent delays separating learning and testing and order of wake and sleep conditions counterbalanced). Adults showed a gain of approximately 10 milliseconds in RTs to legal versus illegal transitions after sleep compared with a nearly 13-millisecond decline in the wake condition. Although children showed an initial gain of 20 milliseconds in their RT to legal versus illegal transitions as compared to adults, there was no additional benefit of sleep with children losing almost half of the original 48-millisecond effect. Furthermore, unlike adults, children's initial learning effect remained stable over waking time.

The effects of sleep on declarative memory consolidation are more closely aligned in children and adults. In a sleep-wake condition, children (9–12 years) learned a minimum of 20 responses to paired associates from a list of 40 word pairs immediately before nighttime sleep; they were tested in the morning and again later in the day after a delay matching their usual nighttime sleep.[99] In a wake-sleep condition the same children learned another list of word pairs in the morning, were tested later in the day after a period of time corresponding to their usual nighttime sleep, then again the following morning after an equivalent delay (with order of sleep-wake and wake-sleep conditions counterbalanced). There was no measurable improvement in performance after time awake but, like adults,[100] children showed improvement after sleep regardless of whether sleep occurred immediately after learning or after time awake. Consistent with adults, the percentage of time spent in NREM sleep correlated positively with gains in memory performance, underscoring continuity in the role of sleep in declarative memory consolidation in children and adults.

A third study investigated the role of sleep in procedural and declarative memory in the same group of children and adults.[101] Children (6–8 years) and adults were tested in a design in which sleep and wake conditions were counterbalanced with an 11-hour interval between training and test. Declarative memory was tested using a word-pairs associate task (adults learned 40 word pairs to a 60% criterion of accuracy; children achieved the same criterion for 20 word pairs) and a task requiring subjects to learn the spatial locations of 15 cards with pictures of animals and everyday objects (to a criterion of 40% correct responses in children and 60% correct responses in adults). The procedural SRT task was more simple than the one used by Fischer and colleagues[98] involving 4 locations instead of 6, with each location cued by a star showing up on 1 of 4 horizontally placed boxes on a computer screen and with each location predicted uniquely by the previous one (eg, 4-1-3-2-4 for the wake condition and 2-3-1-4-2 for the sleep condition). In the declarative memory tasks, degree of retention was indicated by the difference between accuracy at the end of learning and accuracy after the retention interval, whereas in the procedural learning task, retention was indicated by the number of correct key presses to the sequence in the last three 30-second trials at learning versus the three 30-second trials after the retention interval. The benefits of sleep for declarative memory were comparable for children and adults (for word pairs, memory improved with sleep compared with remaining stable over wake; for object location, memory was preserved to a greater degree with sleep than across wake). Although children showed some benefit of sleep on the procedural memory task, the gain was much smaller after sleep than after wake, whereas adults enjoyed a larger gain with sleep than with wake.

Thus, across a range of declarative and procedural memory tasks and a range of ages in childhood, the benefits of sleep on declarative memory consolidation appear to be stable for children and adults, whereas sleep-dependent consolidation of procedural memories undergoes developmental change. This change may stem from greater hippocampal competition in children in whom hippocampally related consolidation of explicit knowledge of the sequence may have interfered with consolidation of procedural learning,[101] especially given that as reported by the investigators children exhibited substantially more verbal encoding of the task in terms of verbally numbering the sequential locations.

Another possibility is that learning may be more susceptible to forgetting during sleep when it is still in a fragile state. Compared with learning in the declarative memory tasks, based on familiar vocabulary and objects and perhaps more easily encoded, children had no prior experience with the SRT task and unlike adults failed to reach asymptote in their learning. Finally, it may be that key aspects of procedural memory consolidation are more likely to take place during wake as opposed to sleep in childhood development. A study investigating the effects of interference on procedural learning in children and adults supports this interpretation.[102] In this study, 9-, 12-, and 17-year-old children learned a 4-finger tapping sequence (eg, 4-1-3-2-4), and 2 hours later, learned a different sequence (eg, 4-2-3-1-4). The experimenters were interested in knowing whether daytime consolidation was differentially susceptible to interference in children and adults. Gains in consolidation of the sequence over 24 hours were significantly reduced in adolescents aged 17 years after learning the second sequence as compared with a condition in which subjects learned no interference sequence. In contrast, 9- and 12-year-old children experienced no reduction in performance as a result of subsequent interference learning, suggesting that children may be less susceptible to interference over waking time than adults, thereby partially explaining the documented gains in children's procedural motor skill learning.

Finally, work with infants also shows effects of sleep on learning. In an early study, 3-month-old infants formed a memory of a particular mobile in one learning experience and their memories were reactivated several weeks later.[103] Retention at test 8 hours after reactivation was correlated with the amount of sleep the infants had during that interval, demonstrating the effect of sleep on consolidation in very young infants.

In a more recent study, 15-month-old children were familiarized with an artificial language while playing quietly with an experimenter in their homes and were tested 4 hours later in the laboratory.[104] (A few example sentences from the artificial language were vot-kicey-jic, pel-wadim-rud, pel-thusev-rud, and vot-wiffle-jic.) A nap group was scheduled at a time of day when they were likely to sleep in the interval between familiarization and test. A no-nap group was scheduled at a time when they were not likely to sleep. It was possible to acquire 2 types of knowledge on exposure to the artificial language: (1) the first word in a sentence predicts the last word; or (2) vot predicts jic and pel predicts rud. The first type of knowledge takes the form of a rule that can be applied to novel sentences, whereas the second type pertains only to sentences identical to those encountered during familiarization.

At test, listening times were obtained to sets of sentences preserving the relationship between the first and third words (eg, vot-kicey-jic, pel-wa-dim-rud, etc) versus sentences violating these relations (eg, vot-kicey-rud, pel-wadim-jic, etc). Children in the no-sleep group showed veridical memory of the strings as reflected in longer looking times to strings preserving the nonadjacent dependencies from familiarization versus strings violating these dependencies, the same as children who were tested immediately after familiarization.[105] In contrast, children in the sleep group listened longer to whichever string type they heard on the first test trial, tracking that particular nonadjacent relation for the remainder of the test trials (16 total). This pattern of listening time behavior was taken as evidence that children applied their knowledge of the dependency rule to novel configurations of the strings (when the string in the first test trial violated the nonadjacency relation from familiarization, infants nevertheless tracked that relation for the remainder of the test trials).

Whether such abstraction was the result of forgetting the stimulus detail or some other abstraction process is not yet known, but the fact that the infants were able to apply their knowledge to strings that were similar but not identical to familiarization strings suggests that with sleep they are able to apply the rule fairly flexibly, an ability that is crucial for young learners. This effect was replicated in a later study in which a sleep and a no-sleep group were tested 24 hours later instead of 4 hours later.[106] The group that slept in the 4-hour interval after familiarization showed the abstraction effect, whereas the group that did not sleep in the interval after familiarization showed no retention the next day. Thus, unlike children and adults who can retain what they have learned until they sleep at night 15-month-old infants appear to need to sleep in an interval soon after learning.

A similar effect shows up in young zebra finches that show deterioration in their newly learned song after sleep during periods of rapid learning.[107] Each day the zebra finches in this study improved with practice on exposure to adult song, with each night resulting in some deterioration. One hypothesis is that the reduction in song structure exhibited after sleep is a way of striking a balance between consolidation and plasticity. If young animals are able to consolidate learning experiences verbatim, they may prematurely commit to learning of a particular structure, whereas if learning deteriorates on a regular basis, they can use the song they produce in the morning (which may manifest some deterioration but not to beginning levels) as a match to the target so that their song will ultimately match the most reliable structures in their input. Such a pattern of advances and retreats protects the learner from overcommitting to any spurious structures produced in their song or gleaned from their input and is supported by the fact that the zebra finches showing the greatest night-to-morning deterioration were the ones who eventually achieved the highest match to adult song. A by-product of sleep-associated forgetting is the ability to apply prior learning to slightly different learning scenarios, as demonstrated by Gomez and colleagues[104,106] in 15-month-old human children.

SUMMARY

Taken together, work examining sleep variables and sleep regulation as predictors of cognitive outcomes, work showing that sleep restriction results in reduced learning compared to normal sleep, and work comparing consolidation of memory across sleep and wake states paints a picture of an essential role for sleep in learning. Children who experience less sleep or less-efficient sleep generally have poorer cognitive and academic outcomes, whereas children who experience experimentally reduced sleep show deficits in higher-level cognitive functioning. Furthermore, studies comparing memory consolidation in wake and sleep states show that sleep is fundamentally implicated in declarative memory consolidation and in the abstraction and retention of rules.

This literature also reveals differences in the effects of sleep in children and adults, with children showing different patterns of sleep-related procedural memory consolidation compared with adults. However, children and adults are similarly affected by reduced sleep in that higher-level cognitive functions are more affected than lower-level functions. And, correlation of poor sleep with poor cognitive outcomes is generally consistent across developmental age, with the caveat that the youngest children may be more affected by reduced sleep than older children[91] and the fact that children who experience less sleep early in childhood may be affected over the long-term, years after they achieve an adequate sleep schedule.[47]

Remaining questions have to do with the extent to which developmental effects in memory and learning may be related to developmental transitions in sleep and whether sleep plays a special role in critical periods of learning. The following are instances of such questions. Are types of learning during infancy influenced and accomplished through the developmental trajectory and ontogeny of sleep? How are different types of learning affected by sleep state? And, when and for what type of memory are naps no longer needed after learning? The future holds the answer to these and many other questions regarding the relationship between sleep and learning in childhood.

ACKNOWLEDGMENTS

The authors thank Sara Viator and Denise Werchan for help with the literature search on which this article is based.

REFERENCES

1. Bonnet MH, Arand DL. We are chronically sleep deprived. Sleep 1995;18(10):908–11.
2. Kopasz M, Loessl B, Hornyak M, et al. Sleep and memory in healthy children and adolescents - a critical review. Sleep Med Rev 2010;14(3):167–77.
3. Wolfson AR, Carskadon MA. Sleep schedules and daytime functioning in adolescents. Child Dev 1998;69(4):875–87.
4. Diekelmann S, Born J. The memory function of sleep. Nat Rev Neurosci 2010;11(2):114–26.
5. Walker MP, Stickgold R. Sleep, memory, and plasticity. Annu Rev Psychol 2006;57:139–66.
6. Stickgold R. How do I remember? Let me count the ways. Sleep Med Rev 2009;13(5):305–8.
7. Sadeh A. Consequences of sleep loss or sleep disruption in children. Sleep Med 2007;2(3):513–20.
8. Frank MG, Issa NP, Stryker MP. Sleep enhances plasticity in the developing visual cortex. Neuron 2001;30(1):275–87.
9. Sengelaub DR. Neural development. In: Nadel L, Goldstone R, editors. Encyclopedia of cognitive science, vol. 3. London (UK): Nature Publishing Group/Macmillan Publishers Limited; 2002. p. 253–61.
10. Graben S, Browne J. Sleep and brain development. Newborn Infant Nurs Rev 2008;8:173–9.
11. Fukushima K, Morokuma S, Nakano H. Significance of fetal behavioral studies [review]. The Ultrasound Obstet Gynecol 2006;6(3-4):172–8.
12. Dan B, Boyd SG. A neurophysiological perspective on sleep and its maturation. Dev Med Child Neurol 2006;48(9):773–9.
13. Kleitman N. Basic rest-activity cycle - 22 years later. Sleep 1982;5(4):311–7.
14. de Weerd AW, van den Bossche RA. The development of sleep during the first months of life. Sleep Med Rev 2003;7(2):179–91.
15. Lombroso CT. Neonatal polygraphy in full-term and premature infants: a review of normal and abnormal findings. J Clin Neurophysiol 1985;2(2):105–55.
16. Stockard-Pope J, Werner S, Bickford RG, et al. Atlas of neonatal electroencephalography. New York: Raven Press; 1992.
17. Anders TF, Keener MA, Kraemer H. Sleep-wake state organization, neonatal assessment and development in premature infants during the first year of life. II. Sleep 1985;8(3):193–206.
18. Ednick M, Cohen AP, McPhail GL, et al. A review of the effects of sleep during the first year of life on cognitive, psychomotor, and temperament development. Sleep 2009;32(11):1449–58.
19. Ellingson RJ, Peters JF. Development of EEG and daytime sleep patterns in low risk premature infants during the first year of life: longitudinal observations. Electroencephalogr Clin Neurophysiol 1980;50(1–2):165–71.
20. Roffwarg HP, Muzio JN, Dement WC. Ontogenetic development of human sleep-dream cycle. Science 1966;152(3722):604–19.
21. Iglowstein I, Jenni OG, Molinari L, et al. Sleep duration from infancy to adolescence: reference values and generational trends. Pediatrics 2003;111(2):302–7.
22. Carskadon MA, Vieira C, Acebo C. Association between puberty and delayed phase preference. Sleep 1993;16(3):258–62.
23. Seo WS, Sung HM, Lee JH, et al. Sleep patterns and their age-related changes in elementary-school children. Sleep Med 2010;11(6):569–75.
24. Taillard J, Philip P, Coste O, et al. The circadian and homeostatic modulation of sleep pressure during wakefulness differs between morning and evening chronotypes. J Sleep Res 2003;12(4):275–82.
25. Carskadon MA. Patterns of sleep and sleepiness in adolescents. Pediatrician 1990;17(1):5–12.
26. Jenni OG, Achermann P, Carskadon MA. Homeostatic sleep regulation in adolescents. Sleep 2005;28(11):1446–54.
27. Reghunandanan V, Reghunandanan R. Neurotransmitters of the suprachiasmatic nuclei. J Circadian Rhythms 2006;4:2.
28. Borbely AA. A two process model of sleep regulation. Hum Neurobiol 1982;1(3):195–204.
29. Curcio G, Ferrara M, De Gennaro L. Sleep loss, learning capacity and academic performance. Sleep Med Rev 2006;10(5):323–37.
30. Taras H, Potts-Datema W. Sleep and student performance at school. J Sch Health 2005;75(7):248–54.

31. Hack M, Taylor HG, Drotar D, et al. Poor predictive validity of the Bayley scales of infant development for cognitive function of extremely low birth weight children at school age. Pediatrics 2005;116(2): 333–41.

32. Borghese IF, Minard KL, Thoman EB. Sleep rhythmicity in premature infants: implications for development status. Sleep 1995;18(7):523–30.

33. Scher A. Infant sleep at 10 months of age as a window to cognitive development. Early Hum Dev 2005;81(3):289–92.

34. Dearing E, McCartney K, Marshall NL, et al. Parental reports of children's sleep and wakefulness: longitudinal associations with cognitive and language outcomes. Infant Behav Dev 2001; 24(2):151–70.

35. Freudigman KA, Thoman EB. Infant sleep during the first postnatal day: an opportunity for assessment of vulnerability. Pediatrics 1993;92(3):373–9.

36. Emde RN, Koenig KL, Wagonfel S, et al. Stress and neonatal sleep. Psychosom Med 1971;33(6):491–7.

37. Scher MS, Steppe DA, Banks DL. Prediction of lower developmental performances of healthy neonates by neonatal EEG-sleep measures. Pediatr Neurol 1996;14(2):137–44.

38. Arditi-Babchuk H, Feldman R, Eidelman AI. Rapid eye movement (REM) in premature neonates and developmental outcome at 6 months. Infant Behav Dev 2009;32(1):27–32.

39. Gertner S, Greenbaum CW, Sadeh A, et al. Sleep-wake patterns in preterm infants and 6 month's home environment: implications for early cognitive development. Early Hum Dev 2002;68(2):93–102.

40. Denenberg VH, Thoman EB. Evidence for a functional role for active (REM) sleep in infancy. Sleep 1981;4(2):185–91.

41. Montgomery-Downs HE, Gozal D. Snore-associated sleep fragmentation in infancy: mental development effects and contribution of secondhand cigarette smoke exposure. Pediatrics 2006; 117(3):e496–502.

42. Beckwith L, Parmelee AH Jr. EEG patterns of preterm infants, home environment, and later IQ. Child Dev 1986;57(3):777–89.

43. Holditch-Davis D, Belyea M, Edwards LJ. Prediction of 3-year developmental outcomes from sleep development over the preterm period. Infant Behav Dev 2005;28(2):118–31.

44. Cohen SE, Parmelee AH, Sigman M, et al. Antecedents of school problems in children born preterm. J Pediatr Psychol 1988;13(4):493–507.

45. Becker PT, Thoman EB. Rapid eye movement storms in infants: rate of occurrence at 6 months predicts mental development at 1 year. Science 1981;212(4501):1415–6.

46. Hayes M. Methodological issues in the study of arousals and awakenings during sleep in the human infants. In: Salzarulo PF, editor. Awakening and sleep—wake cycle across development. Amsterdam (The Netherlands): John Benjamins; 2002. p. 21–45.

47. Touchette E, Petit D, Seguin JR, et al. Associations between sleep duration patterns and behavioral/cognitive functioning at school entry. Sleep 2007; 30(9):1213–9.

48. Buckhalt JA, El-Sheikh M, Keller P. Children's sleep and cognitive functioning: race and socioeconomic status as moderators of effects. Child Dev 2007; 78(1):213–31.

49. El-Sheikh M, Buckhalt JA, Keller PS, et al. Child emotional insecurity and academic achievement: the role of sleep disruptions. J Fam Psychol 2007; 21(1):29–38.

50. Geiger A, Achermann P, Jenni OG. Association between sleep duration and intelligence scores in healthy children. Dev Psychol 2010;46(4):949–54.

51. Lack LC, Wright HR, Bootzin RR. Delayed sleep phase disorder. Sleep Med Clin 2009;4:229–39.

52. Sadeh A, Gruber R, Raviv A. Sleep, neurobehavioral functioning, and behavior problems in school-age children. Child Dev 2002;73(2):405–17.

53. Steenari MR, Vuontela V, Paavonen EJ, et al. Working memory and sleep in 6-to 13-year-old schoolchildren. J Am Acad Child Adolesc Psychiatry 2003;42(1):85–92.

54. Kahn A, Vandemerckt C, Rebuffat E, et al. Sleep problems in healthy preadolescents. Pediatrics 1989;84(3):542–6.

55. Fredriksen K, Rhodes J, Reddy R, et al. Sleepless in Chicago: tracking the effects of adolescent sleep loss during the middle school years. Child Dev 2004;75(1):84–95.

56. Buckhalt JA, El-Sheikh M, Keller PS, et al. Between children's sleep and cognitive functioning: the moderating role of parent education. Child Dev 2009;80(3):875–92.

57. Allen RP. Social factors associated with the amount of school week sleep lag for seniors in an early starting suburban high school. Child Dev 1992; 80:875–92.

58. Cortesi F, Giannotti F, Mezzalira O, et al. Circadian type, sleep patterns, and daytime functioning in adolescence: preliminary data on and Italian representative sample. J Sleep Res 1997;26:707.

59. Giannotti F, Cortesi F, Sebastiani T, et al. Circadian preference, sleep and daytime behaviour in adolescence. J Sleep Res 2002;11(3):191–9.

60. Link SCaA-I S. Sleep and the teenager. J Sleep Res 1995;24:184.

61. Eliasson A, King J, Gould B. Association of sleep and academic performance. Sleep Breath 2002; 6(1):45–8.

62. Drake C, Nickel C, Burduvali E, et al. The pediatric daytime sleepiness scale (PDSS): sleep habits and

school outcomes in middle-school children. Sleep 2003;26(4):455–8.

63. Shin C, Kim J, Lee S, et al. Sleep habits, excessive daytime sleepiness and school performance in high school students. Psychiatry Clin Neurosci 2003;57(4):451–3.

64. Urschitz MS, Guenther A, Eggebrecht E, et al. Snoring, intermittent hypoxia and academic performance in primary school children. Am J Respir Crit Care Med 2003;168(4):464–8.

65. Guilleminault C, Winkle R, Korobkin R, et al. Children and nocturnal snoring: evaluation of the effects of sleep related respiratory resistive load and daytime functioning. Eur J Pediatr 1982; 139(3):165–71.

66. Blunden S, Lushington K, Kennedy D, et al. Behavior and neurocognitive performance in children aged 5–10 years who snore compared to controls. J Clin Exp Neuropsychol 2000;22(5):554–68.

67. Ali NJ, Pitson D, Stradling JR. Sleep disordered breathing: effects of adenotonsillectomy on behaviour and psychological functioning. Eur J Pediatr 1996;155(1):56–62.

68. Blunden S, Lushington, et al. Neuropsychological and psychosocial function in children with a history of snoring or behavioral sleep problems. J Pediatr 2005;146(6):780–6.

69. Archbold KH, Giordani B, Ruzicka DL, et al. Cognitive executive dysfunction in children with mild sleep-disordered breathing. Biol Res Nurs 2004; 5(3):168–76.

70. Beebe DW, Wells CT, Jeffries J, et al. Neuropsychological effects of pediatric obstructive sleep apnea. J Int Neuropsychol Soc 2004;10(7):962–75.

71. O'Brien LM, Mervis CB, Holbrook CR, et al. Neurobehavioral implications of habitual snoring in children. Pediatrics 2004;114(1):44–9.

72. Kurnatowski P, Putynski L, Lapienis M, et al. Neurocognitive abilities in children with adenotonsillar hypertrophy. Int J Pediatr Otorhinolaryngol 2006; 70(3):419–24.

73. Gottlieb DJ, Chase C, Vezina RM, et al. Sleep-disordered breathing symptoms are associated with poorer cognitive function in 5-year-old children. J Pediatr 2004;145(4):458–64.

74. Montgomery-Downs HE, Crabtree VM, Gonzal D. Cognition, sleep and respiration in at-risk children treated for obstructive sleep apnoea. Eur Respir J 2005;25:336–42.

75. O'Brien LM, Mervis CB, Holbrook CR, et al. Neurobehavioral correlates of sleep-disordered breathing in children. J Sleep Res 2004;13(2):165–72.

76. Kaemingk KL, Pasvogel AE, Goodwin JL, et al. Learning in children and sleep disordered breathing: findings of the Tucson Children's Assessment of Sleep Apnea (tuCASA) prospective cohort study. J Int Neuropsychol Soc 2003;9(7):1016–26.

77. Emancipator JL, Storfer-Isser A, Taylor HG, et al. Variation of cognition and achievement with sleep-disordered breathing in full-term and preterm children. Arch Pediatr Adolesc Med 2006;160:203–10.

78. Gozal D. Sleep-disordered breathing and school performance in children. Pediatrics 1998;102(3 Pt 1): 616–20.

79. Richards W, Ferdman RM. Prolonged morbidity due to delays in the diagnosis and treatment of obstructive sleep apnea in children. Clin Pediatr (Phila) 2000;39(2):103–8.

80. Stradling JR, Thomas G, Warley AR, et al. Effect of adenotonsillectomy on nocturnal hypoxaemia, sleep disturbance, and symptoms in snoring children. Lancet 1990;335(8684):249–53.

81. Carskadon MA, Harvey K, Dement WC, Acute restriction of nocturnal sleep in children. Percept Mot Skills 1981;53(1):103–12.

82. Carskadon MA, Harvey K, Dement WC. Sleep loss in young adolescents. Sleep 1981;4(3):299–312.

83. Fallone G, Acebo C, Arnedt JT, et al. Effects of acute sleep restriction on behavior, sustained attention, and response inhibition in children. Percept Mot Skills 2001;93(1):213–29.

84. Randazzo AC, Muehlbach MJ, Schweitzer PK, et al. Cognitive function following acute sleep restriction in children ages 10–14. Sleep 1998;21(8):861–8.

85. Biggs SN, Bauer KM, Peter J, et al. Acute sleep restriction does not affect declarative memory in 10-year-old girls. Sleep Biol Rhythms 2010;8:222–5.

86. Dahl RE. The regulation of sleep and arousal: development and psychopathology. Dev Psychopathol 1996;8(1):3–27.

87. Drummond SP, Brown GG. The effects of total sleep deprivation on cerebral responses to cognitive performance. Neuropsychopharmacology 2001;25(Suppl 5):S68–73.

88. Horne JA. Human sleep, sleep loss and behavior - implications for the prefrontal cortex and psychiatric-disorder. Br J Psychiatry 1993;162:413–9.

89. Jones K, Harrison Y. Frontal lobe function, sleep loss and fragmented sleep. Sleep Med Rev 2001;5(6): 463–75.

90. Fallone G, Acebo C, Seifer R, et al. Experimental restriction of sleep opportunity in children: effects on teacher ratings. Sleep 2005;28(12):1561–7.

91. Sadeh A, Gruber R, Raviv A. The effects of sleep restriction and extension on school-age children: what a difference an hour makes. Child Dev 2003;74(2):444–55.

92. Cousins Hasler J. The effect of sleep extension on academic performance, cognitive functioning and psychological distress in adolescents [doctoral dissertation]. Tucson(AZ): Psychology, The University of Arizona; 2008.

93. Gomez RL. Variability and detection of invariant structure. Psychol Sci 2002;13(5):431–6.

94. Saffran JR, Newport EL, Aslin RN, et al. Incidental language learning: listening (and learning) out of the corner of your ear. Psychol Sci 1997;8(2):101–5.

95. Saffran JR, Johnson EK, Aslin RN, et al. Statistical learning of tone sequences by human infants and adults. Cognition 1999;70(1):27–52.

96. Fiser J, Aslin RN. Unsupervised statistical learning of higher-order spatial structures from visual scenes. Psychol Sci 2001;12(6):499–504.

97. Fiser J, Aslin RN. Statistical learning of new visual feature combinations by infants. Proc Natl Acad Sci U S A 2002;99(24):15822–6.

98. Fischer S, Wilhelm I, Born J. Developmental differences in sleep's role for implicit off-line learning: comparing children with adults. J Cogn Neurosci 2007;19(2):214–27.

99. Backhaus J, Hoeckesfeld R, Born J, et al. Immediate as well as delayed post learning sleep but not wakefulness enhances declarative memory consolidation in children. Neurobiol Learn Mem 2007;89(1):76–80.

100. Plihal W, Born J. Effects of early and late nocturnal sleep on priming and spatial memory. Psychophysiology 1999;36(5):571–82.

101. Wilhelm I, Diekelmann S, Born J. Sleep in children improves memory performance on declarative but not procedural tasks. Learn Memory 2008;15(5):373–7.

102. Dortberger S, Adi-Japha E, Karni A. Reduced susceptibility to interference in the consolidation of motor memory before adolescence. PLoS One 2007;2(2):e240.

103. Fagen JW, Rovee-Collier C. Memory retrieval: a time-locked process in infancy. Science 1983;222(4630):1349–51.

104. Gomez RL, Bootzin RR, Nadel L. Naps promote abstraction in language-learning infants. Psychol Sci 2006;17(8):670–4.

105. Gomez R, Maye J. The developmental trajectory of nonadjacent dependency learning. Infancy 2005;7(2):183–206.

106. Hupbach A, Gomez RL, Bootzin RR, et al. Nap-dependent learning in infants. Dev Sci 2009;12(6):1007–12.

107. Deregnaucourt S, Mitra PP, Feher O, et al. How sleep affects the developmental learning of bird song. Nature 2005;433(7027):710–6.

Sleep States and Memory Processing in Rodents: A Review

Carlyle Smith, PhD

KEYWORDS
- Sleep states • Memory • Slow-wave sleep • REM sleep
- Animals

Many of the early studies examining the relationship between sleep states and memory were done using rats or mice. These studies focused on rapid eye movement (REM) sleep because it seemed to be the most likely candidate to be involved in postacquisition memory processing. Experiments usually involved 1 of the 2 basic techniques. One method was to sleep record the animals (using electroencephalography [EEG]) both before and after task acquisition to observe the changes in sleep parameters. The findings using this method were highly consistent, and most studies reported observing REM sleep increases after successful task acquisition.[1–6] Another method was to deprive the organism of REM sleep for several hours after the end of training and then retest at some later time. A large proportion of the earlier studies involved mechanical REM deprivation (REMD) because it was simple and cheap. Many studies used the "swimming pool" technique, whereby the animal was placed on a pedestal of limited size over water. The animals could get non-REM (NREM) sleep or slow-wave sleep (SWS), which did not require complete muscle relaxation, but they could not achieve the complete muscle atonia of REM sleep without falling from the perch into water.

There has been some criticism of the swimming pool method as being stressful and thus responsible for the impaired performance of animals when they are retested.[7,8] However, there are a significant number of studies that have used alternate nonstressful REMD methods, with identical results. REMD using drug injection,[9–11] mild touching of the animal when REM sleep onset is detected,[12] and gentle head lifting[13] are all examples of low-stress REMD methods that have again provided evidence of REM sleep involvement in memory processing. It is also important to note that there are no alternative studies demonstrating that stress, rather than REM sleep loss, is the important variable contributing to memory loss. Ignoring the many well-done studies over the last 40 years that used this REMD technique, especially those using short (2–4 hours) REMD times, is to dismiss a great deal of important information. Although attempts to reduce stress should always be encouraged, it would be shortsighted to conclude that the many initial REMD studies are of no value.[14] There are many valid studies that can provide an excellent base for more technologically advanced experiments. As stated in an earlier review,[3] the processing of relevant information is possible during REM sleep. New conditioned associations can be formed, and previously learned information can be processed. Also, the material processed during REM sleep can be transferred to the waking state and expressed in behavior. The conclusions reached based on animal studies in the mid-1990s were that the dynamic processes occurring during postlearning REM sleep can contribute to the effectiveness of memory processing and facilitate memory retrieval.[2,3,15] These ideas continue to be supported by more recent animal research. This review concentrates on the more recent animal findings, but the reader should be aware that many useful and informative studies have already been done in this area.

Department of Psychology, Trent University, 1600 West Bank Drive, Peterborough, Ontario K9J 7B8, Canada
E-mail address: csmith@trentu.ca

Sleep Med Clin 6 (2011) 59–70
doi:10.1016/j.jsmc.2010.12.001

REM SLEEP AND MEMORY

One of the basic assumptions of memory consolidation in rodents that has persisted for many years is the idea that memory consolidation takes place within the first few hours of sleep after posttraining acquisition. The REM sleep observed in the first few hours after learning has long been considered to be the most important time for further memory processing, and most studies have not recorded beyond the first 3 to 6 hours. Results of many studies support this view, and recent EEG recording and REMD studies have confirmed these early findings. However, in some studies, EEG recording was continued for several days, and a more complex picture emerged. Not all posttraining REM sleep episodes during the 24-hour period seemed to be involved with memory consolidation. There were only certain posttraining times when the REM sleep duration increased above normal levels. Also, when animals were deprived of REM sleep at these delayed postacquisition times, they showed memory deficits on retest. When REMD was applied outside of these times, there was no memory loss. The special REM periods were named REM sleep windows (RSWs) and their latency to onset and duration seemed to depend on the strain and type of animal being trained, the type of task, and even the number of training trials per session. Massed training induced more extensive posttraining REM sleep than did an equal number of training trials distributed over several days. For extremely distributed trials (5 days), there was a significant increase in REM sleep, which preceded the insight performance of the rat by 24 hours. In this case, the increase in REM sleep duration predicted the improved behavior of the animal. Conversely, when the same strain was trained and exposed to small periods of REMD, it was clear that only short 4-hour periods of REMD were needed to impair the memory for the task when retest took place either the next day or the next week. These studies are unique in that sleep recording was continuous (24 hours per day) and lasted for periods of 8 to 9 days. RSWs have been established for a variety of tasks, including appetitive, aversive, and spatial tasks.[2,14]

Although many of the earlier REM sleep deprivation studies were done using the swimming pool method, a series of more recent studies were done examining the role of the transmitter acetylcholine (ACh) during the RSW.[10] Rats were trained in an 8-arm radial maze spatial task for 10 days, and different groups were exposed to either mechanical REM sleep deprivation via the traditional swimming pool method or given systemic injections of the anticholinergic agent scopolamine at different doses. Rats deprived of REM during the previously established RSW for this task (0–4 hours after training) had inferior learning scores compared with controls that were REM deprived from 4 to 8 hours after the end of the training session or saline controls. There was a dose-dependent increase in the inferior performance for the scopolamine groups injected immediately after the daily training sessions. The larger the dose, the poorer was the learning curve. Performance of rats injected outside of the RSW, so that the scopolamine was active from 4 to 8 hours after training, did not differ from that of saline controls.

In a second study,[11] rats were again trained in the radial maze and given injections of scopolamine bilaterally into the dorsal striatum of test animals immediately after the daily training session. The striatum was chosen because it was considered to be the brain area primarily involved with the "win-stay" version of the maze.[16] As before, scopolamine injections to test rats during the 0- to 4-hour RSW impaired learning progress compared with saline controls and scopolamine control animals injected outside of the RSW (drug active from 4–8 hours after the training session).

These studies support the idea of a time-limited RSW mechanism that enhances the consolidation process. It is also consistent with earlier studies that have found the striatum to be important for the win-stay version of the 8-arm radial maze as well as implicating cholinergic mechanisms previously observed in other REM sleep–dependent tasks.[9]

Although the earlier recording studies were done using visually scored EEG, the shuttle avoidance task has recently been replicated using 50 trials per day for 2 days as the training regime.[17] The source of animal subjects was different, the light-dark cycle timing was modified, and an automated EEG recording system was used, but otherwise everything else was identical. Animals were recorded continuously, and the sleep stages were again visually scored. However, it was possible using an automated scoring system (polygraphic recording analyzer [PRANA], PhiTools, Strasbourg, France) to examine the fine electrical activities taking place in both REM and SWS in more detail. A 17- to 20-hour posttraining RSW was found for rats that were successful learners of the task (60% avoidances or better) when compared with nonlearning controls.[18] The slight changes in the timing of the appearance of the RSW (from an onset at 9 hours posttraining to an onset of 17 hours posttraining) observed in earlier work[17] were attributed mainly to the slightly different strain of the rat and, to a lesser extent, the modest changes in light-dark times with respect to training. The increases were most pronounced in the 17- to 20-hour time period and were clearly caused by an increased number of REM episodes rather than an increase in REM sleep duration. Increases in both theta and beta power occurred during this 17- to 20-hour RSW. During the next 4-hour period (21–24 hours), spindle density (number/minute) and sigma power were increased, whereas SWS was decreased in the learning group. There were no sleep changes on posttraining day 2. Rats that could not learn the task did not show any sleep changes, except for a larger amount of SWS during the 21- to 24-hour period after training on day 1.[18] Results were generally consistent with earlier findings.[17]

These RSW data[18] show an increase in theta during REM followed by increased spindle densities consistent with a 2-stage model of consolidation as has recently been proposed.[19]

Increases in postlearning sleep spindles have also been reported in rats after associative learning (odor-reward pairing task).[20]

THE REM SLEEP GENERATOR

The pedunculopontine nucleus (PPN) and adjacent deep mesencephalic reticular nuclei (DpMe) have been implicated in the generation of REM sleep.[21–23] The rostral PPN is largely composed of glutamatergic cells,[24] whereas the caudal area is almost completely composed of cholinergic neurons.[25] Receptors for the inhibitory transmitter γ-amino butyric acid (GABA) also seem to be involved in REM sleep regulation at the PPN, and the $GABA_B$ agonist baclofen has been shown to significantly reduce REM sleep at this site.[26]

In a recording study,[18] after 24 hours baseline recording, animals were trained on the 2-way shuttle box avoidance task for 50 trials per day over 2 days and retested on day 3. EEG was recorded continuously. Rats were injected with the $GABA_B$ agonist baclofen or saline into the PPN/DpMe region to coincide with the start of a known RSW. Compared with saline control groups, baclofen-injected rats failed to learn the task. PPN/DpMe infusions of the inhibitory $GABA_B$ agonist baclofen decreased REM and impaired subsequent memory performance. Results were consistent with previous work In finding that REM sleep was markedly reduced. Normal GABAergic transmission in the PPN/DpMe seems necessary for REM to occur and for the efficient consolidation of incentive learning.[27]

Datta[28] examined the brainstem activity of the rat and recorded the P wave from cells in the PPN area. In rats, the P wave is comparable to the pontine component of the ponto-geniculo-occiptial wave in the cat, which occurs just before the onset of REM sleep and throughout the REM period. This technique, therefore, allows the direct recording of brainstem cells believed to generate the phasic activity of REM sleep. Rats were trained in a 2-way shuttle avoidance task with regular EEG as well as P-wave activity recorded after task acquisition. There was a 25% increase in REM sleep and a 180% increase in the transitional sleep (tS-R) state between NREM and REM. Also, there was a marked increase in P-wave activity during tS-R and REM sleep, suggesting that P-wave activity modulates cognitive activity. The many connections of this brainstem area to brain structures that are involved in learning are consistent with this idea. In other work, connections to the hippocampus (HP) have been established from the PPN/DpMe. Lesions of CA3 cells impaired memory for the task, whereas P-wave generation and the quality of REM sleep were unchanged. Alternatively, the lesions of CA1 and the dentate gyrus did not interfere with the postsleep memory of the task.[29]

Although no learning task was involved, one group[30] has examined the coordination of HP networks during REM sleep using multiple electrode recording. The group reported significantly higher dentate/CA3 theta and gamma synchrony during REM. On the other hand, gamma power in CA1 and CA1–CA3 gamma coherence showed decreases in REM sleep. These patterns were believed to typify tonic REM sleep. However, phasic bursts in the dentate as well as CA1 neurons were also reported. Phasic REM was characterized by higher theta and gamma synchrony among dentate, CA3, and CA1 neurons. The data suggested enhanced dentate processing but limited CA3-CA1 coordination during tonic REM sleep. In contrast, phasic bursts of activity in REM might provide opportunities to synchronize the HP dentate–CA3-CA1 loop and increase output to cortical targets. The group hypothesized that tonic REM sleep may support off-line mnemonic dentate processing, whereas phasic bursts during REM could promote memory consolidation in the cortex.[30]

MEMORY ENHANCEMENT

Several studies with rats have documented experimental manipulations that enhance memory above normal levels. These studies provide convincing alternative evidence of the existence of memory mechanisms that are active during sleep states, especially REM sleep.

Using an avoidance task, rats were trained to avoid a foot shock when a mild ear (pinna)–conditioned stimulus was presented. During subsequent

REM sleep, the test animals were given the ear stimulations again as reminders of the task. Retesting showed these animals to be superior to rats stimulated during NREM sleep and normally rested nonstimulated animals.[31,32]

One group has reported enhancing memory for a shock-motivated Y-maze discrimination task. Different groups of rats were given either carbachol injections directly into the brainstem pontis oralis area or REM-inducing peptide (eg, corticotropin-like intermediate peptide) intracerebroventricularly after Y-maze training. Rats showed superior memory for the task when compared with saline controls. Experimental rats also showed larger amounts of REM sleep. A third group was exposed to REMD and then trained such that their posttraining sleep contained more REM sleep as a result of REM rebound from the deprivation. These animals were also reported to show superior task memory compared with controls.[32]

Drug-induced enhancement of memory for a shuttle avoidance task has also been reported.[33] It was shown that artificially increasing the P-wave activity by microinjection of carbachol into the P-wave–generating cells enhanced subsequent memory for the task. Selective REM sleep deprivation impaired memory for the shuttle avoidance task, but this impairment was nullified if the rats received a microinjection of carbachol, a cholinergic agonist. P-wave cell lesions resulted in a large reduction in P waves but not in the number of minutes of REM sleep. Compared to control animals, these rats showed no sign of post-REM sleep improvement in shuttle avoidance performance, although initial learning was comparable.

The above-mentioned studies, focusing mainly on REM sleep, add considerable support to the sleep-memory hypothesis, indicating that REM sleep is an important posttraining time for efficient memory consolidation. Furthermore, the phasic portion of REM sleep may well be an important component necessary for efficient memory consolidation. Also, some of the recent RSW studies support the idea of the involvement of SWS as well as REM sleep.

SWS AND MEMORY

Although REM sleep has been extensively studied for many years, the role of SWS in animals has not been as thoroughly explored. Giuditta and colleagues[34] were among the first investigators to argue for a more comprehensive role for memory consolidation that would include both SWS and REM sleep. Since then, SWS has emerged as an important sleep state for memory consolidation.

The HP has been established as a brain region crucial for the encoding and consolidation of memory, particularly declarative memories.[35–38] Long-term potentiation (LTP) remains one of the most popular models of synaptic plasticity.[39–41] The brain area most examined with respect to this model has been the HP. EEG recording from the HP reveals that the primary frequency during active waking and REM sleep is theta. More irregular activity is observed during restful waking and SWS. Recordings from the stratum pyramidale during SWS reveal a ripple oscillation.[42] This event has also been called the sharp wave (SPW) and is basically the same phenomenon measured from the stratum lacunosum.[43] Ripples reflect a large burst discharge of many pyramidal neurons in the HP. The ripple is composed of high-frequency (200 Hz) transient bursts of CA1 pyramidal cells that last 30 to 200 ms and occur during periods of SWS and behavioral immobility.[44,45] These waves are believed to be necessary for the formation and maintenance of memory representations in the neocortex by means of HP-neocortical dialog.[46] Direct suppression of SPWs after the acquisition of an HP-dependent spatial memory task, the 8-arm radial maze, resulted in impaired memory for the task.[47]

SWS AND REPLAY

Extensive work has been done on the CA1 pyramidal cells of the HP. It has been known for some time that these place cells show specificity to the unique location of the rodent in space, with different cells firing at different locations.[48] These cells have been reported to exhibit an experience-dependent reactivation during sleep that is representative of previous waking behavior. Pavlides and Winson[49] performed one of the pioneer studies in this area. They continuously recorded the firing of pairs of CA1 place cells in freely moving rats that did not have overlapping fields. They carefully exposed the rats to areas where one of the cells was active during waking but the other was not. Then during subsequent sleep, they observed increased firing of cells that had been active during waking compared with the inactive cell members of the pairs. These cells appeared to exhibit reactivation during subsequent SWS and REM sleep. There were increased firing rates, along with the greater number of multiple spike bursts and shorter interspike intervals within the burst.

Wilson and McNaughton,[50] using multiple electrode recording sites in the CA1 area of the HP, exposed rats to training in a circular maze. They compared the firing patterns of the neurons in the encoding phase of the task with posttraining SWS as well as SWS before training. They noted cells that had shown highly correlated activity during learning and compared the intercorrelations of their activity to that in posttraining SWS as well as in SWS before the learning experience. It was observed that the correlation patterns in post-SWS were much more similar to those observed during acquisition than they were to the patterns in pretraining SWS. The time frame of this post-SWS activity was short, being strongest in the first 10 minutes of SWS and fading at times beyond 30 minutes. This finding was extended and refined by Kudrimoti and colleagues.[51] A closely associated EEG event, generally referred to as the ripple, is highly correlated in time with the reactivation event. An examination of the times when ensemble reactivation occurs in SWS after training indicates that the event is highly synchronized in time with the occurrence of ripples. Alternatively, reactivation has a very low probability of occurrence during ripple "quiet" times.[51]

Siapas and Wilson[52] tested the hypothesis that the replay phenomenon should be present in the neocortex as well as the HP if this phenomenon represents true memory consolidation. They demonstrated the existence of high temporal correlations between HP ripples and cortical spindles as well as single neuron activity in these 2 brain structures.

The replay phenomenon has been examined in terms of its rate of replay.[53] Replay of place cell neural sequences corresponding to different behavioral locations was found to occur at a faster rate than during the initial behavior, during subsequent SWS. It was observed that there was an approximate 20-fold compression of the original behavioral sequence, which occurred during the subsequent SWS. This phenomenon was not observed in the SWS before the spatial learning.

One of the predictions from this work was that because there is undoubtedly a HP-neocortical dialog, the replay phenomenon should manifest in the cortex in some form as well. Furthermore, this cortical replay should be related to the replay observed in the HP. Such seems to be the case. Ji and Wilson[54] recorded both EEG and individual cell activity from both HP and visual cortices in rats. Recordings were taken during a pretraining sleep session, while they ran in a figure-8 maze, and during the subsequent postsleep period. It was observed that during the posttraining SWS, there were episodes of synchronized multiunit activity from the various cell levels of the visual cortex. These episodes were alternated with decreases in multiunit activity characteristic of cortical cell activity, which typically exhibits alternating "up" and "down" states. Thus, 80 to 300 ms "down" or quiet periods were alternated with increased cellular activity that lasted for several seconds.

These active periods were termed frames and occurred with equal frequency in both presleep and postsleep episodes. The postframes were slightly shorter but exhibited higher firing rates compared with the preframes. The interframe silent periods were correlated with the positive peaks of EEG K-complexes from layer 5 of the cortex. The correlation of cortical frame occurrence with K-complexes, a major component of slow frequency (0.8 Hz) activity, implied that slow oscillations might provide the basic structure for frame production. HP cells have not been so carefully characterized in terms of these up and down states, but fluctuating periods of intensity as frames of multiunit activity from CA1 cells were observed as well. Although there were an equal number of preframes and postframes, HP frames were shorter than cortical frames and had longer interframe silent periods. They had slightly higher firing rates at postframes compared with preframes. The HP frames were correlated with ripples, which almost always appeared within active frames of activity and not during interframe silent periods. A frame could be temporally correlated with one or several ripples, which suggested that the ripple events were triggered by frame activity. Frame onset and offset activity between cortex and HP were also significantly correlated, indicating general activity patterns in these structures reflected an interaction between them during SWS. The activity in the cortex tended to slightly precede that of the HP in time.

These fine temporal replay patterns occurred in both the cortex and HP. The visual cortical cells involved in visual perception during maze running were reactivated during SWS. There seemed to be a difference between the 2 brain areas in terms of the character of the replay. The rats used in the recording study had already had considerable learning experience in the maze. Thus, despite a pretraining SWS condition, it is possible that there was replay because of previous training from several days before the last maze trials. This phenomenon could explain the presence in cortical cells of significantly similar replay activity before the most recent training period. This phenomenon was not as robust from HP cell recording during the presleep condition. On the other hand, both cortical and HP groups showed high-order replay of the recent maze run during post-SWS episodes. This observation is consistent with the idea of the

HP being a temporary and the cortex a more permanent substrate for long-term memory storage.

That the replay during SWS from both brain areas was similar to that of the waking maze-run event led the investigators to conclude that the cortical-HP interaction model of memory formation was supported. It was hypothesized that the cortical frame activation initiated the conditions for replay by activating the HP frames (because their onset precedes that of the HP cells). Sequence memories were then reactivated during ripple events within HP frames. These replayed memories were then sent back to the cortex for more permanent storage as part of a 2-way interaction process between the cortex and the HP.

REM SLEEP AND REPLAY

As mentioned earlier, Pavlides and Winson[49] performed one of the pioneer studies in this area. They found evidence of replay during both SWS and REM sleep. The progression of technology soon led to the possibility of observing larger ensembles of these place cells, and several studies (see SWS section) were performed, which observed the replay of neural ensembles during subsequent SWS, suggesting that SWS reactivation can drive synaptic changes and effect memory consolidation. Replay during SWS, but not REM sleep, was reported. However, Poe and colleagues[55] used a circular maze with multiple reward sites and trained rats to go to these areas for food reward. All animals were recorded using electrode arrays to record place cell activity from multiple cells in the CA1 region both during training and when asleep after the training session. The cell spikes were analyzed in relation to the waking and REM sleep theta-phase activity. During waking, all cells tended to fire in synchrony with the waking theta peaks. However, during subsequent REM sleep, there was a marked difference between the timing of place cells corresponding to familiar maze track areas and cells firing in response to new novel track locations. Cells that responded to familiar track areas tended to fire in a cluster that was coincident with the trough of the background theta. On the other hand, the cells corresponding to novel track regions fired in a cluster that coincided with the theta wave peaks. A time-course study of one animal over a 7-day period showed that there was a gradual transition in cell behavior as the rat became familiar with the track. At first, the place cells fired in clusters coincident with the REM-sleep theta peaks, but as the track became familiar, the cells fired more and more out of

phase with theta peaks until near the end of the week when their activity was coincident with the REM theta troughs. These results were interpreted in terms of LTP mechanisms. Because the HP is known to have a finite number of neurons compared with the neocortex, it was reasoned that although the maze experience was novel and new, the postlearning REM sleep was involved with LTP processes in the HP. As the track became more familiar, the information was transferred to other brain areas, and the HP was in the process of erasing this redundant information to make room for more new material.

Louie and Wilson,[56] using the same experimental situation, exposed rats to the circular maze (10–15 minutes session), and then allowed them 1 to 2 hours of sleep. This procedure was repeated for several days. They observed temporally sequenced ensemble firing rate patterns reflecting several seconds to several minutes of behavior. Then, during subsequent REM sleep, they observed a replay of these cell ensembles with sequence and timing preserved. The reproduction of this ensemble firing occurred on a time scale that was approximately the same as the waking behavior or perhaps slightly slower. Thus long temporal sequences of patterned multineuronal activity were observed to be replayed during REM sleep. A modulated pattern of local field potential theta frequency power (6–10 Hz) during waking was observed, which was closely coupled with the task experience, with bursts of increased activity after each trial in the maze. This observation was correlated with the theta in subsequent REM so as to correspond with the neuronal replay. The REM theta peak power values were significantly larger than the theta power of the troughs, suggesting that theta oscillation modulation observed during waking was also represented during REM sleep. It was noted that preexperience sleep recording (recording beginning on a new test day 24 hours later) in this study showed that these cell assembly replays were still in evidence. Thus there would seem to be a long-term persistence of these replay episodes, longer than that expected and observed from SWS. The investigators suggested that a connection to prefrontal cortical areas may be needed to help organize the temporal order for the HP with respect to behavior. Earlier studies did not find any REM sleep replay activity.[51] However, the recording times for cell assembly sequences for these studies were in milliseconds to seconds rather than seconds to minutes, and the sequences observed by Louie and Wilson[56] took place over a relatively much longer period. The exact role of the theta rhythm is not known yet.

EMOTIONAL MEMORY

Memories of an emotional nature have been a component of many rodent sleep studies. Avoidance paradigms have often used negative incentives such as shock. Generally, the involvement. of REM sleep has been observed both from recording studies and selective REMD studies. In earlier studies, memory loss was reported if REMD was imposed after task acquisition, and REM sleep increases were observed in animals that were allowed normal sleep after task acquisition. There are several reviews of these studies.[1,2]

A few more recent studies have attempted to identify the brain structures involved with fear conditioning. In one study, auditory tones were paired with foot shock during waking in rats. Cells from the medial geniculate (MGB) and lateral amygdala (LA) were recorded during waking and then during subsequent REM sleep. Neuronal activity quickly increased in both cell groups during awake conditioning. Then, when the rats were allowed to sleep, the training tone was presented again during REM sleep at a level that did not awaken the rats. In previously conditioned rats, both MGB and LA cells increased their firing rates in response to the tone. A pseudoconditioned group did not show these cellular changes either during wakefulness or sleep. Furthermore, the level of neuronal activity in each animal during wakefulness was highly correlated with the level of activity induced during subsequent REM sleep. It was concluded that enhanced activity in MGB and LA reflected emotional learning–induced neuronal plasticity.[57,58]

In a contextual fear study, rats were exposed to both contextual and cued fear conditioning. Groups of rats were deprived of REM sleep from 0 to 5 hours or from 5 to 10 hours after the conditioning experience. REMD was found to result in memory loss for the contextual situation in the 0- to 5-hour window but not in the 5- to 10-hour window. Cued fear was not disrupted by REMD at any posttraining time. The HP-dependent contextual fear conditioning was disrupted, whereas the cued fear, dependent on both HP and amygdala, was spared. It was concluded that REMD selectively impairs HP-dependent memory, leaving amygdala-dependent memories intact.[59]

In a recent study, using a step-down task, it was reported that there were no REM sleep increases in the 6 hours after training. In fact, there was a drop in the REM sleep percentage. EEG recording directly from the basolateral amygdala (BLA) and central amygdala (CeA) nuclei indicated that there was related activity in these areas. Generally, BLA activity was increased, whereas CeA activity was decreased. These results are in agreement with the previous study that cued fear conditioning, involving the amygdala, does not seem to be REM dependent.[60] However, it may be premature to assume that a reduction in REM sleep does not reflect memory consolidation. REM sleep may be involved in a way that is not yet understood. Similar REM sleep results were reported in rats after fear conditioning involving the pairing of light with inescapable foot shock. There was a decrease in the number of REM episodes, average duration of episodes, and percentage REM.[61]

There is much more research to be done before the relationship between REM sleep, emotional memory consolidation, and the brain structures involved is understood.

NEUROCHEMICAL AND GENETIC FACTORS

The understanding of the relationship between sleep and memory at the molecular level is just beginning to build momentum. There is a substantial amount of information on the biochemical nature of the states of sleep and even more is known about memory processes alone. However, the interaction of these 2 important activities is not well understood. There are several transmitters that are believed to be involved with memory consolidation. These transmitters include ACh, norepinephrine (NE), serotonin (ie, 5-hydroxytryptamine [5-HT]), dopamine, glutamate, and adenosine and GABA.

There is general agreement that the waking brain shows high levels of 5-HT, NE, and ACh. During NREM sleep, the levels of ACh are low, whereas that of NE and 5-HT are also low but much higher than ACh. During REM sleep, the levels of ACh are again very high, whereas NE and 5-HT levels drop to very low levels.[62]

ACh

One transmitter that has received some attention in the sleep-memory context is ACh. In an animal study,[9] rats were exposed to the 2-way shuttle avoidance task with a well-established RSW between 9 to 12 hours after the end of training. Different groups of rats were given systemic injections of the protein synthesis inhibitor anisomycin such that the substance would be active during the RSW or at control times several hours before or after the RSW. Only rats with the protein inhibitor active during the RSW showed memory loss for the task on retest. Furthermore, analysis of both the levels of ACh and the enzyme acetylcholine esterase showed that the inhibitor had suppressed activity in groups at all of the times compared with saline controls. It was concluded that ACh was necessary for memory processing at the RSW, but not at times outside of the 9- to 12-hour posttraining RSW. Similar behavioral results were observed with the ACh agonist, scopolamine.[9] Using the Morris water maze spatial task and the conditioned cue preference task, similar results were reported at unique RSWs using scopolamine.[14]

More recently, Legault and colleagues[10] showed that systemic injections of scopolamine interfered with the consolidation of a radial arm maze task when injected to coincide with the posttraining RSW, but not at other posttraining times. In further work, it was shown that direct injections of scopolamine into the striatum were effective at blocking consolidation during the same RSW but not at other posttraining times.[10] Thus, several animal studies, using different tasks, strongly suggest that ACh is active in memory consolidation processes at certain posttraining times during REM sleep. As mentioned earlier, other investigators have showed memory enhancement, one group using the ACh agonist carbachol to enhanced P-wave activity[33] and another showing enhanced memory for a Y-maze discrimination task.[32]

Intracellular Mechanisms

Although most transmitter systems have not been extensively studied in relation to sleep states and memory consolidation, the potential and scope for future studies involving these transmitters and their subsequent intracellular consequences seems promising.[63] For example, increased levels of ACh and decreased levels of 5-HT could trigger a cascade via G protein–coupled receptors. Subsequent changes in the second messenger cyclic adenosine monophosphate (cAMP) and activation of protein kinase A and cAMP response element–binding protein (CREB) could enhance memory consolidation in structures such as the HP.[64,65] Some initial studies have been done.

One group[66] studied the expression of the immediate early gene zif-268. The expression of this gene is triggered by sustained membrane depolarization, N-methyl-D-aspartate channel opening, and calcium influx. This system implicates the transmitter glutamate. Rats were sleep recorded and exposed to the informal learning situation of an enriched environment (EE) for 3 hours. The controls were kept in a more restricted environment. Different groups were sacrificed during subsequent waking, NREM, or REM sleep and their brains were examined for changes in zif-268 expression. The levels of zif-268 dropped from waking to NREM to REM sleep in the controls.

However, in the animals present in EE, zif-268 levels dropped during NREM sleep, but increased again during REM sleep, indicating that the learning situation resulted in increased gene expression during subsequent REM sleep. The brain areas most involved appeared to be the striatum and amygdala.[67]

In other studies, these investigators examined the effects of unilateral high-frequency stimulation of the rat HP during waking on gene expression.[68] This procedure is known to result in LTP, a model of synaptic plasticity.[39] Measuring the same gene, they observed that compared with waking, the stimulated hemisphere showed a drop in zif-268 expression during NREM sleep, but an increase again during REM sleep. By contrast, the control hemisphere showed a steady drop from waking to NREM to REM sleep, providing additional evidence of gene reinduction during REM sleep after a relevant waking experience. Furthermore, they showed that the HP activity during poststimulation REM sleep was essential for REM-associated zif-268 activity in the cortex and amygdala. Using the same paradigm, they extended these findings, examining zif-268 as well as secondary gene activation. They found that 11 genes were enhanced in the LTP hemisphere of rats that were allowed to sleep, with HP and prefrontal cortices showing the greatest activity.[69]

Ribeiro and colleagues[70] examined the changes during waking, SWS, and REM sleep of extracellular neuronal activity, local field potentials, and expression levels of plasticity-related immediate early genes (IEG) Arc and zif-268 in rats exposed to a novel spatio-tactile experience. Analyses were performed on the HP and somatosensory cortex (SC). At the electrical recording level, increased firing rates were observed during post-experience SWS, but they only lasted for minutes in the HP, whereas they persisted for several hours in the SC. IEG expression was upregulated in the SC but not in the HP during REM sleep, 4 hours after the novel experience for both Arc and zif-268, with Arc expression being stronger. Arc expression in the cortex showed a significant correlation with local field potential amplitudes in the spindle range of 10 to 14 Hz. The investigators concluded that memories of the waking novel experience were reactivated during SWS and consolidated during REM sleep in a 2-step consolidation process.

Datta's group[71,72] examined the role of CREB, a transcription factor that plays a role in long-term memory formation. Using the 2-way shuttle avoidance task, the group observed, as previously mentioned, an increase in brainstem P-wave density as a result of successful learning. In addition, an increased activation of CREB activity in the cells of the dorsal HP (DH) was shown. This activity was most prominent in the CA3 subfield of the HP, with lesser activity in the CA1 and dentate gyrus areas. The activity was most pronounced 3 hours after the end of training, which coincided with the peak P-wave intensity previously observed. Most recently, this group has reported that the P-wave generator is directly involved in the molecular events of the DH and the amygdala after successful 2-way shuttle avoidance acquisition. The P-wave generator increased phosphorylation of CREB and expression of *Arc* protein as well as the mRNA of *Arc*, *BDNF*, and *Egr-1* in the DH and amygdala. Selective lesioning of the generator, without reducing time spent in tonic REM sleep, reduced expression of these molecules and resulted in impaired task memory after training. Increased expression of these molecules was observed after direct cholinergic stimulation of the P-wave generator. Results support the idea that P-wave generation is an important factor in postacquisition REM sleep for memory enhancement. Furthermore, the activation of P-wave–generating cells may provide a glutamatergic-activating stimulus to the HP and amygdala for the neuronal activation–dependent gene expression and protein synthesis that are necessary for the cognitive functions of the DH and amygdala.[72]

STATUS OF SLEEP-MEMORY THEORIES

Theories concerning the relationship between sleep states and memory processes have not kept up with the fast pace of new information. However, it seems clear that attributing memory processing activity to a single sleep state[2,73,74] gives way to more complex multiple stage theories. In light of the literature, a comprehensive theory would have to include both SWS and REM sleep, with attention to the subcategories and architectural detail for each of these states. The slow oscillations, activity at other frequencies (such as theta, sigma), and spindles of SWS as well as the tonic and phasic components of REM sleep should be included. Although the different types of memory (declarative vs nondeclarative) have not been a major focus in animal studies, the different types of tasks might well induce different subsequent sleep patterns. Clearly, the HP-cortical connection will be a part of any new theory, but some learning may induce different sleep responses (such as those reported after tasks with a large emotional component). Certainly, a clearer understanding of the complex electrophysiologic activity at the neuronal level should also be included. A comprehensive theory also should adequately describe the many neurochemical intracellular activities that occur in the brain during sleep after successful learning and how they relate to memory consolidation. Although no such theory exists at this time, its development would help explain the many new findings as well as allow some precise predictions about further studies.

FUTURE DIRECTIONS

Rodent data that have accumulated over the last 15 to 20 years add considerably to the early conceptualizations of how sleep states are involved with memory consolidation. Technological advances have allowed experiments that more carefully define the nature of sleep states to postacquisition memory processing. Studies that can include electrophysiologic, neurophysiologic, neurochemical, and behavioral variables in a single experiment will provide particularly compelling data.

The timing of postsleep consolidation times must eventually be addressed. Most experiments now examine sleep changes within the first 3 to 6 hours after acquisition. Although this focus will undoubtedly result in a better understanding of how memories are formed, it is clear that memory processing during sleep endures for many days after the end of training. Examination of these longer-term events will have to be explored as well.

The extent to which electrophysiologic and neurochemical changes occur during sleep may vary considerably between behavioral tasks as well as between species and strain of the organism being studied. Different amounts of training on the same task can provide variable postsleep responses. Similar behavioral tasks and animal strains between laboratories should be encouraged.

REFERENCES

1. Smith C. Sleep states and learning: a review of the animal literature. Neurosci Biobehav Rev 1985;9: 157–68.
2. Smith C. Sleep states, memory processes and synaptic plasticity. Behav Brain Res 1996;78:49–56.
3. Hennevin E, Hars B, Maho C, et al. Processing of learned information in paradoxical sleep: relevance for memory. Behav Brain Res 1995;69:125–35.
4. McGrath MJ, Cohen DB. REM sleep facilitation of adaptive waking behavior: a review of the literature. Psychol Bull 1978;85:24–57.
5. Pearlman C. REM sleep and information processing: evidence from animal studies. Neurosci Biobehav Rev 1979;3:57–68.
6. Fishbein W, Gutwein BW. Paradoxical sleep and memory storage processes. Behav Biol 1977;19: 425–64.

7. Siegal JM. The REM sleep-memory consolidation hypothesis. Science 2001;294:1058–63.

8. Vertes R. The case against sleep and memory consolidation. Behav Brain Sci 2000;23:867.

9. Smith C, Tenn C, Annett R. Some biochemical and behavioral aspects of the paradoxical sleep window. Can J Psychol 1991;45:115–24.

10. Legault G, Smith C, Beninger RJ. Scopolamine during the paradoxical sleep window impairs radial arm maze learning in rats. Pharmacol Biochem Behav 2004;49:715–21.

11. Legault G, Smith C, Beninger R. Post-training intrastriatal scopolamine or flupenthixol impairs radial maze learning in rats. Behav Brain Res 2006;170: 148–55.

12. Ishikawa A, Kanayama Y, Matsumara H, et al. Selective rapid eye movement deprivation impairs the maintenance of long-term potentiation in the rat hippocampus. Eur J Neurosci 2006;24:243–8.

13. Datta S, Mavanji V, Ulloor J, et al. Activation of phasic pontine-wave generator prevents rapid eye movement sleep deprivation-induced learning impairment in the rat: a mechanism for sleep dependent plasticity. J Neurosci 2004;24:1416–27.

14. Smith CT. The REM sleep window and memory processing. In: Maquet P, Smith C, Stickgold R, editors. Sleep and brain plasticity. Oxford (UK): Oxford Press; 2003. p. 117–33.

15. Smith C. Sleep states and memory processes. Behav Brain Res 1995;69:137–45.

16. McDonald RJ, White NM. A triple dissociation of memory systems: hippocampus, amygdala and dorsal striatum. Behav Neurosci 1993;107:3–22.

17. Smith C, Lapp L. Prolonged increases in both PS and number of REMS following a shuttle avoidance task. Physiol Behav 1986;36:1053–7.

18. Fogel S, Smith C, Beninger R. Evidence for 2-stage models of sleep and memory: learning-dependent changes in spindles and theta in rats. Brain Res Bull 2009;79:445–51.

19. Smith C, Aubrey JB, Peters KR. Different roles for REM and stage 2 sleep in motor learning: a proposed model. Psychol Belg 2004;44:81–104.

20. Eschenko O, Molle M, Born J, et al. Elevated sleep spindle density after learning or after retrieval in rats. J Neurosci 2006;26:12914–20.

21. Rye DB. Contributions of the pedunculopontine region to normal and altered REM sleep. Sleep 1997;20:757–88.

22. Datta S, Siwek DF, Patterson EH, et al. Localization of pontine PGO wave generation sites and their anatomical projections in the rat. Synapse 1998;30:409–23.

23. Datta S. Neuronal activity in the peribrachial area: relationship to behavioral state control. Neurosci Biobehav Rev 1995;19:67–84.

24. Clements J, Grant SGN. Glutamate-like immunoreactivity in neurons of the laterodorsal tegmental

and pedunculopontine nuclei in the rat. Neurosci Lett 1990;120:70–3.

25. Rye DB, Saper C, Lee H, et al. Pedunculopontine tegmental nucleus of the rat: cytoarchitecture, cytochemistry, and some extrapyramidal connections of the mesopontine tegmentum. J Comp Neurol 1987; 259:483–528.

26. Ulloor J, Mavanji V, Saha S, et al. Spontaneous REM sleep is modulated by the activation of the pedunculopontine tegmental $GABA_B$ receptors in the freely moving rat. J Neurophysiol 2004;19:1822–31.

27. Fogel S, Smith C, Beninger R. Increased GABAergic activity in the region of the pedunculopontine and deep mesencephalic reticular nuclei reduces REM sleep and impairs learning in rats. Behav Neurosci 2010;124:79–86.

28. Datta S. Avoidance task training potentiates phasic pontine-wave density in the rat: a mechanism for sleep-dependent plasticity. J Neurosci 2000;20: 8607–13.

29. Datta S, Saha S, Prutzman SL, et al. Pontine-wave generator activation dependent memory processing of avoidance learning involves the dorsal hippocampus in rat. J Neurosci Res 2005;80:727–37.

30. Montgomery SM, Sirota A, Buzsaki G. Theta and gamma coordination of hippocampal networks during waking and rapid eye movement sleep. J Neurosci 2008;28(26):6731–41.

31. Hars B, Hennevin E, Pasques P. Improvement of learning by cueing during postlearning paradoxical sleep. Behav Brain Res 1985;1:241–50.

32. Wetzel W, Wagner T, Balschun D. REM sleep enhancement induced by different procedures improves memory retention in rats. Eur J Neurosci 2003;18:2611–7.

33. Mavanji V, Datta S. Activation of the pontine-wave generator enhances improvement of learning performance: a mechanism for sleep dependent plasticity. Eur J Neurosci 2003;17:359–70.

34. Giuditta A, Ambrosini MV, Montagnese P, et al. The sequential hypothesis of the function of sleep. Behav Brain Res 1995;69:157–66.

35. Zola-Morgan S, Squire LR, Amaral DG. Human amnesia and the medial temporal region: enduring memory impairment following a bilateral lesion limited to field CA1 of the hippocampus. J Neurosci 1986;6: 2950–67.

36. Zola-Morgan S, Squire LR, Mishkin M. The neuroanatomy of amnesia: amygdala-hippocampus versus temporal stem. Science 1982;218:1337–9.

37. Squire RL, Zola-Morgan S. Memory: brain systems and behavior. Trends Neurosci 1988;11:170–5.

38. Squire LR. Memory and the hippocampus: a synthesis from findings with rats, monkeys and humans. Psychol Rev 1992;99:195–231.

39. Bliss TVP, Lomo T. Long lasting potentiation of synaptic transmission in the dentate area of the

anaesthetized rabbit following stimulation of the perforant path. J Physiol (London) 1973;232:331–56.

40. Ivanco TL, Racine RJ. Long-term potentiation in the reciprocal corticohippocampal and corticocortical pathways in the chronically implanted, freely moving rat. Hippocampus 2000;10:143–52.

41. Pavlides C, Greenstein YJ, Grudman M, et al. Long-term potentiation in the dentate gyrus is induced preferentially on the positive phase of theta-rhythm. Brain Res 1988;439:383–7.

42. O'Keefe J, Nadel L. The hippocampus as a cognitive map. New York: Oxford University Press; 1978.

43. Buzsaki G. Hippocampal sharp waves: their origin and significance. Brain Res 1986;398:242–52.

44. Buzsaki G, Horvath Z, Urioste R, et al. High-frequency network oscillation in the hippocampus. Science 1992;256:1025–7.

45. Chrobak J, Buzsaki G. High-frequency oscillations in the output networks of the hippocampal-entorhinal axis of the freely behaving rat. J Neurosci 1996;16:3056–66.

46. Buzsaki G. The hippocampo-neocortical dialogue. Cereb Cortex 1996;6:81–92.

47. Girardeau G, Benchenane K, Wiener SI, et al. Selective suppression of hippocampal ripples impairs spatial memory. Nat Neurosci 2009;12:1219–21.

48. O'Keefe J, Dostrovsky J. The hippocampus as a spatial map. Preliminary evidence from unit activity in the freely moving rat. Brain Res 1971;34:171–5.

49. Pavlides C, Winson J. Influences of hippocampal place cell firing in the awake state on the activity of these cells during subsequent sleep episodes. J Neurosci 1989;9:2907–18.

50. Wilson MA, McNaughton BL. Reactivation of hippocampal ensemble memories during sleep. Science 1994;265:676–8.

51. Kudrimoti HS, Barnes CA, McNaughton BL. Reactivation of hippocampal cell assemblies: effects of behavioral state, experience and EEG dynamics. J Neurosci 1999;19:4090–101.

52. Siapas AG, Wilson MA. Coordinated interactions between hippocampal ripples and cortical spindles during slow-wave sleep. Neuron 1998;21:1123–8.

53. Lee AK, Wilson MA. Memory of sequential experience in the hippocampus during slow wave sleep. Neuron 2002;36:1183–94.

54. Ji D, Wilson MA. Coordinated memory replay in the visual cortex and hippocampus during sleep. Nat Neurosci 2007;10:100–7.

55. Poe GR, Nitz DA, McNaughton BL, et al. Experience-dependent phase reversal of hippocampal neuron firing during REM sleep. Brain Res 2000;855:176–80.

56. Louie K, Wilson MA. Temporally structured replay of awake hippocampal ensemble activity during rapid eye movement sleep. Neuron 2001;29:145–56.

57. Hennevin E, Maho C, Hars B. Neuronal plasticity induced by fear conditioning is expressed during paradoxical sleep: evidence from simultaneous recordings in the lateral amygdala and the medial geniculate nucleus. Behav Neurosci 1998;112:839–62.

58. Hennevin E. Expression and modulation of memory traces during paradoxical sleep. In: Maquet P, Smith C, Stickgold R, editors. Sleep and brain plasticity. Oxford (UK): Oxford Press; 2003. p. 101–16.

59. Graves LA, Heller EA, Pack AI, et al. Sleep deprivation selectively impairs memory consolidation for contextual fear conditioning. Learn Mem 2003;10:168–76.

60. Mavanji V, Siwek DF, Patterson EH, et al. Effects of passive-avoidance training on sleep-wake state specific activity in the basolateral and central nuclei of the amygdala. Behav Neurosci 2003;117:751–9.

61. Sanford LD, Silvestri AJ, Ross RJ, et al. Influence of fear conditioning on elicited ponto-geniculo-occipital waves and rapid eye movement sleep. Arch Ital Biol 2001;134:81–99.

62. Aston-Jones G, Bloom FE. Activity of norepinephrine-containing locus coeruleus neurons in behaving rats anticipates fluctuations in the sleep-wake cycle. J Neurosci 1981;1:887–900.

63. Graves L, Pack A, Abel T. Sleep and memory: a molecular perspective. Trends Neurosci 2001;24:237–43.

64. Isiegas C, McDonough C, Huang T, et al. A novel conditional genetic system reveals that increasing neuronal cAMP enhances memory and retrieval. J Neurosci 2008;28:6220–30.

65. Vecsey CG, Baille G, Jaganath D, et al. Sleep deprivation impairs cAMP signalling in the hippocampus. Nature 2009;461:1122–5.

66. Ribeiro S, Goyal V, Mello CV, et al. Brain gene expression during REM sleep depends on prior waking experience. Learn Mem 1999;6:500–6.

67. Pavlides C, Ribeiro S. Recent evidence of memory processing in sleep. In: Maquet P, Smith C, Stickgold R, editors. Sleep and brain plasticity. Oxford (UK): Oxford Press; 2003. p. 327–62.

68. Ribeiro S, Mello CV, Velho T, et al. Induction of hippocampal long-term potentiation during waking leads to increased extra-hippocampal *zif-268* expression during ensuing REM sleep. J Neurosci 2002;22:10914–23.

69. Romcy-Pereira RN, Erraji-Benchekroun L, Smryrniotopoulos P, et al. Sleep-dependent gene expression in the hippocampus and prefrontal cortex following long-term potentiation. Phsyiol Behav 2009;98:44–52.

70. Ribeiro S, Shi X, Englehard M, et al. Novel experience induces persistent sleep-dependent plasticity in the cortex, but not in the hippocampus. Front Neurosci 2007;1:43–55.

71. Datta S. Activation of phasic pontine-wave generator: a mechanism for sleep-dependent memory processing. Sleep Biolog Rhyth 2006;4:16–26.

72. Datta S, Li G, Auerbach S. Activation of phasic pontine-wave generator in the rat: a mechanism for expression of plasticity-related genes and proteins in the dorsal hippocampus and amygdala. Eur J Neurosci 2008;27:1876–92.

73. McNaughton BL, Barnes CA, Battaglia FP, et al. Off-line reprocessing of recent memory and its role in memory consolidation: a progress report. In: Maquet P, Smith C, Stickgold R, editors. Sleep and brain plasticity. Oxford (UK): Oxford Press; 2003. p. 225–46.

74. Buzsaki G. Memory consolidation during sleep: a neurophysiological perspective. J Sleep Res 1998;7(Suppl 1):17–23.

A Molecular Basis for Interactions Between Sleep and Memory

Pepe J. Hernandez, PhD*, Ted Abel, PhD

KEYWORDS

- cAMP • PKA • CREB • Learning • Memory • NREM
- REM • Oscillation

The sleep-for-memory hypothesis posits that a primary function of sleep is memory consolidation, the process by which newly acquired information is stabilized and stored. While sleep may serve in other capacities,[1] a growing body of literature detailing the beneficial effects of sleep on memory has given the sleep-for-memory hypothesis considerable momentum. It has been argued that the core function of sleep is likely cellular, because, like the need for sleep, the basic functions of cellular proteins are remarkably consistent across phylogenetic lines, regardless of differences in sleep architecture and brain complexity.[2] Indeed, the molecular mechanisms that mediate memory consolidation are also conserved across species and in light of evidence suggesting that wakeful experience is recapitulated on a cellular level during sleep, it may be that the same molecular processes that promote memory consolidation might also be reengaged during sleep to further stabilize and improve memory.

This article presents several key concepts and molecular processes that are known to underlie learning and memory consolidation. Also, it provides an overview of some of the electrophysiological events specific to various sleep states and might serve to modulate activity within these signaling pathways. Finally, it addresses recent progress, questions still unanswered, and the challenges and limitations associated with the methodologies used to study sleep-memory interactions on a molecular level.

STAGES OF MEMORY PROCESSING

Memory storage is often differentiated into pharmacologically dissociable stages.[3] During the encoding or acquisition phase, perceived information is transformed into synaptic activity through the propagation of electric and chemical signals between neurons at synapses. Changes in synaptic activity resulting from the encoding process must be stabilized or consolidated if they are to become part of an enduring memory. The consolidation process can be further distinguished into 3 forms: synaptic consolidation, which occurs soon after acquisition or encoding; systems consolidation, during which memory is reorganized throughout the brain over weeks to years; and reconsolidation, which stabilizes recently retrieved memories. Often, multiple learning sessions or trials are required to form a particular association and related memory. Therefore, memory of those requiring multiple iterations of acquisition, consolidation, and reconsolidation. Thus, sleep could potentially influence multiple stages of memory processing (**Fig. 1**).[4] This article reviews some of the key molecular events involved in each stage of learning and memory formation, with the idea that some or all

This work was supported by grants from NIA (AG-18199), NIMH (MH-60244), NHLBI (HL-60287), the Whitehall Foundation, the John Merck Foundation and the David and Lucile Packard Foundation (T.A.); NSF (0706858) (P.J.H.).
The authors have nothing to disclose.
Department of Biology, University of Pennsylvania, 433 South University Avenue, Lynch Laboratories, Room 222, Philadelphia, PA 19104, USA
* Corresponding author.
E-mail address: pepej@sas.upenn.edu

Sleep Med Clin 6 (2011) 71–84
doi:10.1016/j.jsmc.2010.12.004

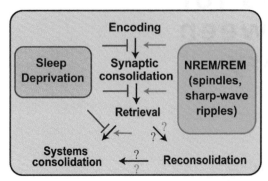

Fig. 1. Permissive and inhibitory effects of sleep and sleep deprivation on the stages of memory formation. Encoding allows relevant environmental information to be converted into a neural construct that can be stored within the brain and recalled at a later time. Newly learned information must be stabilized by strengthening and stabilizing synapses that are activated during learning. Once consolidated, memory can be retrieved and used by the organism. Under certain conditions, retrieved memories render them sensitive to disruption, requiring them to undergo the process of reconsolidation. Reconsolidated and previously learned memories may also be consolidated on a systems level. Systems consolidation typically refers to the reorganization or transference of memory traces out of the hippocampus to areas in the neocortex. Sleep-dependent processing of memory has been shown to affect all stages of memory formation. Neural oscillations during rapid eye movement (REM) and non-REM sleep have permissive enhancing effects on each stage of memory formation (*blue arrows*), whereas sleep deprivation or the prevention of sleep-related oscillations impairs memory formation (*red lines*). The role of sleep and sleep deprivation in reconsolidation is less understood and is denoted with question marks.

the processes described later could potentially be reengaged during sleep-dependent memory processing. **Fig. 2** provides a schematic of the molecular pathways involved in memory consolidation.

Acquisition/Encoding

Many neurotransmitter systems are involved in the encoding process, but the study of glutamate-mediated transmission of information through α-amino-3-hydroxy-5-methyl-4-isoxazolepropionic acid receptors (AMPARs) and N-methyl-D-aspartate receptors (NMDARs) is important in the study of learning and memory and its cellular correlate long-term potentiation (LTP, discussed later).[21,22] Transduction of environmental information through glutamate and other modulatory receptors triggers transcriptional and translational mechanisms that mediate gene expression, synaptic plasticity, and ultimately behavior. Specifically, Ca^{2+} influx

through glutamate receptors can trigger the covalent modification (eg, phosphorylation) of preexisting proteins at active synapses,[23,24] resulting in short-term changes in synaptic strength. These short-term changes, along with changes in the presynaptic neuron, alter the probability of the postsynaptic neuron firing to future stimuli. As shown in **Fig. 2**, activity-dependent increases in intracellular Ca^{2+} levels can activate Ca^{2+}-calmodulin, which can then activate calcium/calmodulin-dependent protein kinase (CaMK) II and protein kinase A (PKA). CaMKII and PKA can then phosphorylate AMPAR and NMDAR subunits thereby altering synaptic transmission. This increase in receptor function is temporary and allows information to be conveyed in the short term. Short-term memory can then be committed to long-term memory (LTM) or forgotten as the synaptic connections eventually weaken.

Two main theories have been proposed to explain how sleep might influence learning and memory formation: the active systems theory and the synaptic homeostasis hypothesis. The active systems theory proposes that cellular activity observed during learning is replayed or recapitulated in some form during postlearning sleep.[25,26] Cellular replay during sleep could mimic the encoding process or help to link new memories to previously consolidated memory networks. According to the synaptic homeostasis hypothesis,[27] the net strength of synapses increases during wake and is downscaled during sleep. Indeed, AMPAR subunit phosphorylation has been shown to be higher during wake and lower after sleep in the cortex and hippocampus of rats[28] (but see[29]). The elimination of synapses that have only undergone weak encoding, and are not needed for LTM formation, could reduce the signal to noise ratio in the brain and allow the encoding of new information to proceed more efficiently. Both theories cite mechanisms that could affect encoding and memory processing and are not necessarily mutually exclusive.

Synaptic Consolidation

Gene transcription and translation is required for the consolidation of LTM[23] and the maintenance of LTP[30]; LTP is the long-lasting enhancement of signal transmission between neurons at synapses that have been repeatedly stimulated. Like short-term memory and LTM, LTP can be distinguished into at least 2 forms: early and late (L-LTP); L-LTP requires transcription and translation. An important aspect of L-LTP is the maintenance of increased synaptic strength brought about by the trafficking of AMPARs

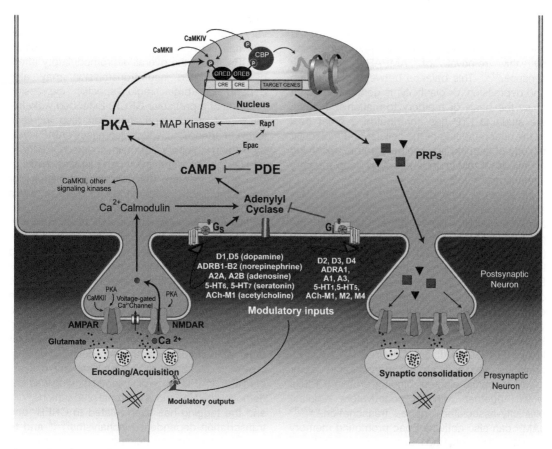

Fig. 2. Signaling pathways involved in the encoding and consolidation of learning and memory. During encoding, presynaptic release of glutamate activates N-methyl-D-aspartate receptors (NMDARs) and α-amino-3-hydroxy-5-methyl-4-isoxazolepropionic acid receptors (AMPARs) in the postsynaptic cell (synapse shown on the left). Ca^{2+} influx through these receptors and voltage-gated Ca^{2+} channels activates Ca^{2+}-calmodulin which can then activate calcium/calmodulin-dependent protein kinase (CaMK) II, protein kinase A (PKA), and other signaling kinases, thereby increasing levels of AMPARs and NMDARs through the phosphorylation of various receptor subunits. Long-term memory formation requires transcription- and translation-dependent mechanisms to strengthen and stabilize synaptic connectivity. Ca^{2+} influx during encoding also activates adenylyl cyclase (AC), which increases intracellular levels of the second messenger cyclic AMP (cAMP). Increased cAMP levels upregulate PKA-dependent phosphorylation of other protein kinases (eg, the MAPKs) that, together with PKA, can translocate to the nucleus to activate the transcription factor cAMP response element binding protein (CREB). cAMP also activates exchange protein directly activated by cAMP (Epac),[5] although the role of Epac in sleep-related plasticity has not been investigated. Signaling proteins such as CaMKIV and CaMKII[6–13] also play a role in CREB activation. CREB together with its coactivator CREB binding protein (CBP) regulates gene transcription by promoting the binding of transcriptional machinery to target genes and by making target genes more accessible to transcriptional machinery by altering chromatin structure.[14–17] Proteins synthesized in the soma or locally in dendrites[18] are transported to synapses that have been tagged by prior activity. AMPAR trafficking into the postsynaptic membrane (shown in the synapse on the right) plays an important role in the long-term maintenance of synaptic strength. Importantly, cAMP signaling can be regulated by the actions of neurotransmitters that bind to G protein–coupled receptors. Levels of modulatory neurotransmitters, many of which are coupled to both stimulatory (G_s) and inhibitory (G_i) G protein–coupled receptors, change dramatically during the sleep-wake cycle. Activation of G_s- and G_i-coupled receptors stimulates and inhibits AC activity, respectively, which alters cAMP production accordingly.[3] Sleep deprivation and circadian rhythms can also alter intracellular levels of cAMP, MAPK, and other plasticity-associated molecules.[19,20] CRE, cAMP response element; PDE, phosphodiesterase; PRPs, plasticity-related proteins. (*Adapted from* Abel T, Nguyen PV. Regulation of hippocampus-dependent memory by cyclic AMP-dependent protein kinase. Prog Brain Res 2008;169:98; with permission.)

containing the GluR1 subunit to the appropriate synapses. Conversely, the strength of synapses can be decreased during synaptic depression by the removal of AMPARs from the synapse.[31,32] This balance between potentiation and depression, or plasticity, is generally thought of as the basis of memory formation.[33] Indeed, the study of LTP has contributed a great deal to the understanding of the cellular and molecular biology of learning and memory and is becoming an important tool in understanding sleep-memory interactions.[30,34,35]

Increases in intracellular Ca^{2+} levels also play a critical role in plasticity-associated transcription and translation. Ca^{2+} influx stimulates the production of the second messenger cyclic AMP (cAMP) by adenylyl cyclase. cAMP activates at least 3 targets important in memory processing: PKA, exchange protein directly activated by cAMP (Epac), and hyperpolarization-activated cyclic nucleotide-gated channels.[36] Once activated, PKA and other plasticity-associated kinases (eg, MAPK, extracellular signal–regulated kinase [ERK], CaMKII, and CaMKIV[8,11]) can phosphorylate and activate the transcription factor cAMP response element binding protein (CREB), which together with its coactivators regulate plasticity-associated gene transcription.[6,37–39] cAMP can also activate Epac promoting memory formation through Rap1 and possibly CREB.[5,40] Plasticity-related proteins (PRPs) are translated and targeted to previously activated synapses that require stabilization. Protein synthesis occurring locally in the dendrites can also be regulated by Ca^{2+} influx through NMDARs and has been shown to play an important role in memory formation.[41]

At least 1 round of transcription- and translation-dependent consolidation is required to stabilize a new memory. However, Bourtchouladze and colleagues[42] and other investigators[43–45] have shown that depending on the training protocol used, 2 or more waves of PKA activation and protein synthesis are required after training.[46–48] The exact nature of these waves of activity is unknown but their existence suggests that some sort of feedback or cyclic activity occurs during the posttraining time, a time when the experimental subjects were likely sleeping.

Fluctuations in the levels of excitatory and inhibitory neurotransmitters occurring during sleep and extended wakefulness can have important influences on memory consolidation.[49,50] For example, sleep-dependent fluctuations of levels of neurotransmitters that bind to G protein–coupled receptors (GPCRs) can stimulate or inhibit adenylyl cyclase to modulate cAMP levels (see **Fig. 2**).

Dopamine and acetylcholine levels are known to vary dramatically during different sleep stages and can activate both stimulatory and inhibitory GPCRs. Thus, the overall neuromodulatory effect of sleep-related neurotransmission may also depend on brain region–specific expression patterns of a particular GPCR. Extended wakefulness and sleep deprivation can also increase levels of adenosine, which decreases cAMP levels by binding inhibitory G protein–coupled GPCRs. In addition, sleep deprivation can increase levels of phosphodiesterase, the enzyme responsible for degrading cAMP, although the mechanism of this increase is still under investigation.[20]

How neurons keep a record of which synapses out thousands are to be strengthened and maintained is an active area of research. Restated from a molecular level perspective, how does encoding at a particular synapse instruct the cell to deliver the required PRPs to that particular synapse during subsequent periods of wake and sleep? To solve this problem, it was proposed that encoding triggers the production or delivery of molecular tags at synapses activated during learning, providing an "address" to facilitate the delivery of PRPs.[51,52] Evidence of synaptic tagging was first demonstrated in various neuronal preparations,[53–56] and the tagging has been related to CREB- and transcription-dependent mechanisms[56,57] and to A kinase–anchoring proteins that serve to compartmentalize PKA in functionally distinct regions of the neuron.[58] The identity of the tags and specific PRPs remain, for the most part, unknown. However, Homer1a has been proposed to fulfill most criteria of a potential tag[59] and is upregulated in mice after sleep deprivation suggesting that there may be a connection between the overall level of activated synapses and tag expression with extended wakefulness.[60] Protein kinase Mζ (zeta) is also thought to be a PRP and plays a role in the maintenance of L-LTP and memory.[61,62] Indeed, any of the cellular machinery involved in local translation might serve as a tag. Importantly, a behavioral correlate of tagging has been described,[63] in which weak inhibitory avoidance training in rats, which does not normally produce LTM for the event, can be consolidated into LTM by exposure to a novel environment. This conversion requires protein synthesis and dopamine (D_1/D_5) receptor activity. In light of these findings, tagging might be a method by which PRPs mobilized during postlearning wake and sleep are targeted to the appropriate synapses.

Because bouts of sleep soon after learning enhance memory,[64] it seems that sleep benefits synaptic consolidation in particular. Sleep can improve speed and reduce errors in motor performance tasks or word recall tasks.[65,66] Whether these benefits are conferred by sleep-specific molecular pathways or boost activity in molecular pathways already activated during wakeful consolidation is not fully understood. The fact that sleep-specific gene expression has been demonstrated could argue for the former possibility but does not exclude the latter. That is, in addition to sleep-dependent modulation of gene expression initiated during learning, sleep-dependent gene expression could occur in parallel.

Systems Consolidation

Once consolidated on a synaptic level, newly formed memories undergo a process of reorganization on a broader systems level. Systems consolidation traditionally refers to the slow transference of memory out of the hippocampus to the neocortex for permanent storage,[67–69] but more current views include mechanisms by which new memories are incorporated into distributed networks of previously consolidated memories.[70] Further, it has been cited that some memories always remain hippocampus dependent and that others have never resided there, stressing the notion that the neocortex is likely more involved during early consolidation than previously appreciated.[71,72] These theories are beginning to bridge the events that occur during synaptic consolidation to those classically defined as systems consolidation,[67] incorporating a role of sleep in both processes.

The sleep-for-memory hypothesis also posits that sleep, in addition to enhancing encoding and synaptic consolidation, promotes the reorganization of memory during systems consolidation. Pharmacologic studies of the function of sleep in systems consolidation are difficult to perform because of the long time course of memory reorganization and the distributed nature of memory traces, but genetic studies in mice[73] and human imaging studies seem to be consistent with a role for sleep in systems consolidation. Using a declarative word-pair learning task, Gais and colleagues[74] showed that sleep after learning increased functional connectivity between the medial prefrontal cortex and hippocampus during retrieval tests 48 hours later and enhanced activity in prefrontal cortex during retrieval 6 months later. Sleep-dependent shifts to neocortex-based memory representations could result in more efficient retrieval.[70,75] A functional magnetic resonance imaging study conducted by Orban and colleagues[76] also demonstrates that sleep promotes the reorganization of brain activity over long periods. The investigators trained human

subjects in a place-finding navigational task; those who slept after training tended to use an extended hippocampo-neocortical network to perform the task in early retrieval sessions and the striatal regions in later sessions. However, subjects who were sleep deprived showed significantly less striatal activity during later retrieval tests, suggesting that sleep deprivation altered the normal course of memory reorganization over time. Interestingly, performance between the 2 groups was unaltered, demonstrating that the reorganization of memory between systems does not always enhance performance in learning and memory tasks but can reflect the transference of well-learned information to systems designed to process automated behaviors.

Retrieval and Reconsolidation

Retrieval refers to the reactivation of memory traces. Under certain conditions, retrieval of a memory trace renders it sensitive to disruption by amnesic treatments for a short period.[77–79] Such sensitized memories require reconsolidation, by which the retrieved memories undergo further consolidation to be restabilized and stored. Reconsolidation could be a mechanism by which older memories are updated and cross-linked with newly formed memories.[80] Although much less is known about the molecular events underlying retrieval and reconsolidation, they seem to have unique molecular signatures involving specific molecular pathways and brain regions.[81–83] However, PKA activity seems to be a consistent requirement for the retrieval and reconsolidation of many forms of memory, at least in some brain regions.[84,85] For example, retrieval of 1-trial inhibitory avoidance memory requires the activation of AMPARs and NMDARs in addition to PKA and ERK in the hippocampus and cortex. However, in the amygdala, only AMPAR activity is required for retrieval; NMDAR activity, PKA, and ERK are unnecessary.[86–88] Although reconsolidation has been demonstrated in humans,[89] there has been much debate on the boundary conditions that dictate whether reconsolidation of a retrieved memory occurs[90] and if amnesia related to the blockade of reconsolidation reflects memory erasure or impaired retrieval.[82] The effect of sleep on retrieval and reconsolidation has been less studied, but sleep may affect the reorganization of memories that undergo reconsolidation (see[70,91] for more detailed reviews on the role of sleep in memory reactivation and reconsolidation). Rapid eye movement (REM) sleep deprivation impairs the retrieval of discriminative avoidance training in rats.[92]

Summary

Memory traces instantiated during wake seem to be altered in a sleep-dependent fashion. Sleep occurring within several hours of training can improve performance in a variety of memory tasks and induce changes in retrieval-associated brain activity,[93,94] suggesting that the neuronal substrates of memory are redistributed during sleep.[95] Initial studies suggest that sleep-dependent plasticity, much like the initial encoding and consolidation of memory, requires the activation of NMDARs, AMPARs, and PKA.[65,96–98] Synaptic tagging and multiple waves of intracellular activity might guide and induce the sleep-related strengthening of memories, respectively. However, it is not entirely clear whether sleep-dependent plasticity is controlled by cellular and molecular events that precede sleep, in a sense priming the trace for further modification during sleep, or whether sleep acts more or less independently on memory. Thus, a primary goal from a molecular standpoint is to determine how the unique properties of the sleeping brain might tap into the molecular mechanisms known to instantiate memories during wake. How sleep might interact with the molecular pathways involved in memory consolidation is examined in the following sections.

SLEEP STATES AND MEMORY

In many organisms, sleep can be broadly characterized as fluctuating between 2 states: REM sleep and non-REM (NREM) sleep.[99] Each of these states may contribute differentially to memory consolidation.[100] Several fundamental oscillatory patterns can be seen in the electroencephalogram (EEG) during wake and sleep, including delta (<1.0–4 Hz), theta (4–9 Hz), beta (15–35 Hz), and gamma (>40 Hz) oscillations.[101] During wake, low-amplitude high-frequency gamma oscillations can be observed throughout the cortex,[102,103] but as the brain transitions from wake to NREM sleep (which has 4 stages in humans), gamma oscillations give way to the characteristic high-amplitude low-frequency slow waves (<4 Hz) of NREM sleep.[104] During REM sleep, rapid desynchronous gamma oscillations are obvious in the cortical EEG as are oscillations in the theta frequency,[105–107] which are similar to theta rhythms observed during exploratory movements performed during wake.[108–112] REM sleep is further characterized by the presence of muscle atonia except for eye and whisker movements in humans and rodents, respectively.[113–116]

Several approaches have been traditionally used to study sleep-memory interactions. As illustrated earlier, sleep deprivation has been a useful tool but can produce unintended effects on learning and memory because it can be stressful on the organism. A second approach correlates sleep-related oscillations (eg, their duration, frequency, phase, and power) to gains in task performance. A third approach examines how learning alters subsequent sleep architecture and EEG patterns. Newer approaches attempt to alter or prevent the occurrence of specific oscillatory rhythms during sleep to provide more direct evidence of sleep-memory interactions. In the following sections, how oscillatory patterns characteristic to NREM and REM sleep might influence plasticity-associated signaling pathways, which are summarized in **Fig. 2**, is further examined. Also, how homeostatic and circadian control of sleep states might influence sleep-memory interactions on a molecular level is discussed.

NREM and Memory

During NREM sleep, slow-wave oscillations in the delta frequency and specialized oscillations known as sleep spindles (11–15 Hz)[117,118] and sharp wave-ripple (SPW-R) complexes (140–200 Hz) can be observed in the hippocampus and neocortex.[112,119,120] Spindle activity during stage 2 NREM correlates well with improvements in memory tasks (see[121] for a detailed review on sleep spindles). Stages 3 and 4 constitute deep sleep and are collectively referred to as slow wave sleep (SWS). Slow waves reflect the synchronous transitions between "up states," during which neurons of the cortex and hippocampus are collectively depolarized and fire together, and "down states," during which they are hyperpolarized and relatively silent.[122] Indeed, evidence suggests that spindles and SPW-Rs play a particularly important role in sleep-memory interactions[123,124] and tend to occur together during SWS.[125–128] This temporal coherence is thought to reflect the coordinated transfer of information between the hippocampus and neocortex[127,129]; however, the exact nature of this hippocampo-neocortical "dialog" is not fully understood on a cellular or molecular level.[123,130,131] Interestingly, the sequence in which specific neurons (eg, place cells in the hippocampus) are activated during wake seems to be recapitulated, or replayed, in various forms during subsequent periods of wake,[132] NREM (in particular during SPW-Rs[26,132]), and REM sleep.[26] Furthermore, blockade of hippocampal output in genetically modified mice impaired systems consolidation and reduced the frequency of hippocampal ripples and experience-dependent ripple-associated reactivation of hippocampal cell pairs.[73]

In light of evidence demonstrating that sequences of neuronal activation observed during learning reoccur during postlearning periods of wake and sleep, it is tempting to hypothesize that there is an ensuing period of molecular replay when molecular events engaged during learning are reengaged during sleep. Several studies support the notion that signaling pathways mediating hippocampal long-term plasticity must be reactivated to consolidate memory, perhaps even for its maintenance as a remote cortex-dependent memory trace.[46,133–135]

Perhaps, the most compelling evidence that sleep-associated oscillations influence memory processing has been obtained from studies in which oscillations have been either enhanced or inhibited after learning. Marshall and colleagues[136] used transcranial electric stimulation in humans to stimulate SWA during NREM sleep after learning in 2 different hippocampus-dependent tasks or 2 procedural motor skill tasks. Stimulation with slow 0.75 Hz oscillations during early night NREM sleep selectively enhanced memory retention in the hippocampus-dependent tasks and increased SWS, as well as endogenous cortical slow oscillations and spindle activity in the frontal cortex, providing the most direct evidence of a role for sleep-associated oscillatory rhythms in memory. Stimulation at 5 Hz or 0.75 Hz late in the night had no enhancing effect relative to sham stimulation. Although memory for the procedural tasks generally benefited from sleep, no further gains were observed with slow-wave stimulation. Another study examined the effect of suppression of SPW-R complexes in rats trained in a hippocampus-dependent spatial reference memory task using the radial arm maze.[137] SPW-R events blocked by stimulation of the ventral hippocampal commissure during postlearning rest and sleep significantly impaired performance relative to rats that received the same number of stimulations but had intact SPW-R events. Lastly, it has been demonstrated that reexposure to olfactory cues during SWS, which were part of a training context in a prior learning task, was found to enhance subsequent memory.[138] Thus, the type and timing of oscillations during NREM sleep may play an important role in sleep-dependent memory consolidation. Despite advances in the understanding of sleep-memory interactions on an electrophysiological level and of the molecular biology of LTM formation, little direct evidence exists to link sleep-related oscillations with memory processing on a molecular level.

REM and Memory

During REM sleep, brain activity in the gamma and theta frequency range is similar to that during wake,[139,140] but the body is paralyzed due to atonia; for this reason, REM is often referred to as paradoxic sleep. REM sleep deprivation can result in memory impairments; however, the degree of impairment seems to be determined by the complexity of the task. Indeed, simple tasks (eg, passive avoidance, one-way active avoidance, and simple mazes), which are quickly learned, are less affected by REM sleep deprivation. Conversely, tasks that require more complex associations to be learned (eg, discriminative and probabilistic learning, complex maze learning, and instrumental conditioning) are particularly sensitive to REM sleep deprivation.[141,142] Furthermore, REM sleep deprivation is effective only if the animal has reached a certain level of learning.[141,143] In humans, the amount of REM sleep late in sleep cycle (and NREM sleep early in the night) correlates with improvements on visual discrimination tasks.[144] Similar results have been found in several tasks and species and have been reviewed in detail elsewhere.[123,124]

On a molecular level, little is known of the effects of REM sleep on memory processing. REM sleep deprivation, however, has been linked to lower binding of noradrenaline to α- and β-adrenergic receptors throughout the brain,[145] which could result in memory impairments by lowering cAMP levels via decreased stimulation of adenylyl cyclase by stimulatory G protein. REM sleep deprivation has also be been linked to low levels of phosphorylated CREB, and deprivation of both NREM and REM sleep for 5 hours has been shown to produce decreased cAMP signaling in the hippocampus accompanied by impairments in the consolidation of contextual fear memory in mice.[20] Thus, cAMP-related signaling also seems to play a role in the effects of REM sleep deprivation on memory consolidation.

HOMEOSTATIC AND CIRCADIAN CONTROL OF SLEEP-DEPENDENT MEMORY PROCESSING

To understand sleep-memory interactions, one must also understand how sleep and synaptic plasticity are regulated by homeostatic and circadian processes. The homeostatic regulation of sleep is observed during increased levels of adenosine during sleep deprivation, changes in gene expression, the posttranslational modification of proteins, and increases in SWS during periods of sleep rebound after sleep deprivation.[146] Importantly, wakeful experience and learning have been shown to increase the length of time spent in NREM and REM sleep.[147] Increased sleep duration due to learning could provide a longer window of time for oscillatory events including spindles and SPW-Rs to occur, thereby increasing the beneficial effects of sleep on memory consolidation. Alternatively, increased sleep duration could accompany learning-dependent alterations in the electrophysiological properties (eg, power) of sleep-associated oscillatory activity. Indeed, learning-dependent increases in sleep need accompanied by increased SWA during NREM sleep and higher numbers of spindles in brain regions activated during learning have been demonstrated and correlated with levels of sleep-dependent performance enhancements.[148–150] Thus, sleep need, at least under certain circumstances, seems to be regulated at local and global levels, warranting further investigation.[151] In contrast, Walker and colleagues[152] have shown that doubling the quantity of initial training does not alter the amount of sleep-dependent learning in a finger-tapping motor task. However, it has been shown that difficult motor sequences benefit more from sleep than easy motor sequences.[153,154] This difference could arise since there may be more room for sleep-dependent improvement of weakly encoded procedural memories. If task performance in well-learned memories is near maximal, as far as accuracy and speed, then little benefit from sleep might be expected.

In associative learning paradigms (eg, fear conditioning), task difficulty might predict the magnitude of postlearning changes in sleep architecture and oscillatory patterns. Indeed, Steenland and colleagues[155] recently examined the effects of trace fear conditioning in which the associative strength between a conditioned stimulus (a tone) and the unconditioned stimulus (a footshock) was altered by changing the difficulty of the task. That is, the task can be made more difficult to learn by lengthening the duration of trace time, the delay between termination of the conditioned stimulus and presentation of the unconditioned stimulus. Mice conditioning using a short 15-second trace resulted in significant enhancements in delta power during subsequent NREM sleep relative to baseline, whereas mice conditioned with a more difficult 30-second trace showed no significant enhancements in delta power relative to baseline. Together, these data suggest that learning and plasticity affect sleep need and the electrophysiological properties of subsequent sleep, which, in turn, can modulate sleep-dependent memory enhancements.

Circadian rhythms, in addition to homeostatic mechanisms, can influence memory processing and postlearning sleep[156] through the regulation of transcription and translation within various brain regions.[157,158] For example, hippocampal gene expression and enzyme activity have been shown to vary over the course of the day.[19,159,160] In fact, up to 10% of the mammalian transcriptome may be under the control of circadian rhythms.[7,161–163] Relevant to the role of the cAMP-PKA-CREB pathway in sleep-memory interactions, Eckel-Mahan and colleagues[19] have shown that ERK, MAPK, and CREB phosphorylation, in addition to cAMP levels, undergo circadian oscillations in the hippocampus. Interference with these oscillations by physiologic and pharmacologic agents impaired the maintenance of hippocampus-dependent LTM, suggesting that the reactivation of the cAMP-CREB pathway is influenced by circadian rhythms.

Clock genes (eg, *Clock, Bmal1, Period, Cryptochrome,* and *Timeless*) are closely related to circadian rhythms in mammals and *Drosophila* and are thought to modulate learning and memory. However, their role in sleep-memory interactions has been largely unexplored.[164,165] A possible function of clock genes is to bind sleep and memory consolidation. For example, clock genes may play a role in the temporally restricted expression of the effects of learning on subsequent sleep (ie, increased slow-wave activity confined to the first few hours of sleep). The activity of clock genes might also explain why sleep can be delayed until later in the same day yet still benefit memory.[152,166–168] Certainly, genetic models targeting clock genes will prove useful in determining their role in sleep-memory interactions.

MOLECULAR REPLAY AND SLEEP-DEPENDENT MEMORY PROCESSING

The replay of hippocampal cellular activity (eg, during ripple events) is thought to reflect cellular activity that occurred during prior bouts of wake.[26,169–172] Therefore, it is possible that cellular replay during sleep could trigger a similar replay of the molecular events that occurred during encoding and early consolidation.[173] Although the notion of molecular replay is far from conclusive, many of the signaling pathways shown in **Fig. 2** function in synaptic plasticity,[9] synaptic homeostasis,[9] learning and memory,[10,12,13] and sleep.[7,174] Indeed, the cAMP-PKA-CREB pathway plays a role in the transduction of environmental information during memory formation and is modulated by sleep deprivation, circadian rhythms, and neurotransmitter systems involved in sleep-wake regulation.[20,174–178] Thus, the cAMP-PKA-CREB signaling pathway is well suited to play an integrative role in sleep-memory interactions.

THE USE OF GENETIC MODELS TO STUDY SLEEP-MEMORY INTERACTIONS

The ability to manipulate gene expression in mice and other organisms is an important tool in understanding sleep.[179] Regional and even cell type–specific expression of altered genes can assess their role within precise loci in the brain. Although the temporal control of gene expression has improved,[180] the required temporal resolution to study sleep-memory interactions in mice, for example, must be on the order of minutes due to rapid sleep-wake transitions. Moreover, rapid regulation is required because most studies are conducted when mice are normally sleeping and return to sleep shortly after training. Without this level of temporal control, genetic modifications could produce nonspecific effects on memory and sleep or alter sleep-wake regulation preventing a direct analysis of sleep-memory interactions. Approaches similar to those used in optogenetic systems, whereby specific cell types can be optically stimulated in vivo via expression of light-activated channel rhodopsins,[181] could be engineered to precisely modulate oscillatory patterns that occur during sleep providing a direct measure of their effects on memory.

SUMMARY

Mounting evidence demonstrates that sleep plays a beneficial role in memory consolidation. Multifunctional signaling pathways involved in memory, sleep, and sleep-wake regulation may have evolved to integrate the effects of sleep with memory processing. However, to better understand the role of sleep in memory processing, the establishment of testable falsifiable hypotheses using a combination of new genetic approaches and methods that regulate the electrophysiological properties of the brain during sleep is needed. These approaches will provide more direct evidence of sleep-memory interactions. This type of evidence would circumvent the correlational confines of standard methodologies moving the field toward a deeper understanding of the molecular basis of sleep-memory interactions.

REFERENCES

1. Palagini L, Rosenlicht N. Sleep, dreaming, and mental health: a review of historical and neurobiological perspectives. Sleep Med Rev Sep 15, 2010. [Epub ahead of print].
2. Cirelli C, Tononi G. Is sleep essential? PLoS Biol 2008;6:e216.
3. Abel T, Lattal KM. Molecular mechanisms of memory acquisition, consolidation and retrieval. Curr Opin Neurobiol 2001;11:180.
4. Walker MP, Stickgold R. Sleep, memory, and plasticity. Annu Rev Psychol 2006;57:139.
5. Ma N, Abel T, Hernandez PJ. Exchange protein activated by cAMP enhances long-term memory formation independent of protein kinase A. Learn Mem 2009;16:367.
6. Ahmed T, Frey JU. Plasticity-specific phosphorylation of CaMKII, MAP-kinases and CREB during late-LTP in rat hippocampal slices in vitro. Neuropharmacology 2005;49:477.
7. Cirelli C, Gutierrez CM, Tononi G. Extensive and divergent effects of sleep and wakefulness on brain gene expression. Neuron 2004;41:35.
8. Enslen H, Sun P, Brickey D, et al. Characterization of Ca2+/calmodulin-dependent protein kinase IV. Role in transcriptional regulation. J Biol Chem 1994;269:15520.
9. Ibata K, Sun Q, Turrigiano GG. Rapid synaptic scaling induced by changes in postsynaptic firing. Neuron 2008;57:819.
10. Kang H, Sun LD, Atkins CM, et al. An important role of neural activity-dependent CaMKIV signaling in the consolidation of long-term memory. Cell 2001; 106:771.
11. Matthews RP, Guthrie CR, Wailes LM, et al. Calcium/calmodulin-dependent protein kinase types II and IV differentially regulate CREB-dependent gene expression. Mol Cell Biol 1994; 14:6107.
12. Wei F, Qiu CS, Liauw J, et al. Calcium calmodulin-dependent protein kinase IV is required for fear memory. Nat Neurosci 2002;5:573.
13. Wu LJ, Zhang XH, Fukushima H, et al. Genetic enhancement of trace fear memory and cingulate potentiation in mice overexpressing Ca2+/calmodulin-dependent protein kinase IV. Eur J Neurosci 1923;27:2008.
14. Vecsey CG, Hawk JD, Lattal KM, et al. Histone deacetylase inhibitors enhance memory and synaptic plasticity via CREB: CBP-dependent transcriptional activation. J Neurosci 2007;27:6128.
15. Levenson JM, Sweatt JD. Epigenetic mechanisms: a common theme in vertebrate and invertebrate memory formation. Cellular and Molecular Life Sciences 2006;63:1009.
16. Swank MW, Sweatt JD. Increased histone acetyltransferase and lysine acetyltransferase activity and biphasic activation of the ERK/RSK cascade in insular cortex during novel taste learning. J Neurosci 2001;21:3383.

17. Wood MA, Hawk JD, Abel T. Combinatorial chromatin modifications and memory storage: a code for memory? Learn Mem 2006;13:241.

18. Sutton MA, Schuman EM. Dendritic protein synthesis, synaptic plasticity, and memory. Cell 2006;127:49.

19. Eckel-Mahan KL, Phan T, Han S, et al. Circadian oscillation of hippocampal MAPK activity and cAMP: implications for memory persistence. Nat Neurosci 2008;11:1074.

20. Vecsey CG, Baillie GS, Jaganath D, et al. Sleep deprivation impairs cAMP signalling in the hippocampus. Nature 2009;461:1122.

21. Kelley AE, Andrzejewski ME, Baldwin AE, et al. Glutamate-mediated plasticity in corticostriatal networks: role in adaptive motor learning. Ann N Y Acad Sci 2003;1003:159.

22. Ortiz O, Delgado-Garcia JM, Espadas I, et al. Associative learning and CA3-CA1 synaptic plasticity are impaired in D1R null, Drd1a-/- mice and in hippocampal siRNA silenced Drd1a mice. J Neurosci 2010;30:12288.

23. Hernandez PJ, Abel T. The role of protein synthesis in memory consolidation: progress amid decades of debate. Neurobiol Learn Mem 2008;89:293.

24. Routtenberg A, Rekart JL. Post-translational protein modification as the substrate for long-lasting memory. Trends Neurosci 2005;28:12.

25. Ji D, Wilson MA. Coordinated memory replay in the visual cortex and hippocampus during sleep. Nat Neurosci 2007;10:100.

26. Wilson MA, McNaughton BL. Reactivation of hippocampal ensemble memories during sleep. Science 1994;265:676.

27. Tononi G, Cirelli C. Sleep function and synaptic homeostasis. Sleep Med Rev 2006;10:49.

28. Vyazovskiy VV, Cirelli C, Pfister-Genskow M, et al. Molecular and electrophysiological evidence for net synaptic potentiation in wake and depression in sleep. Nat Neurosci 2008;11:200.

29. Hagewoud R, Havekes R, Novati A, et al. Sleep deprivation impairs spatial working memory and reduces hippocampal AMPA receptor phosphorylation. J Sleep Res 2010;19:280.

30. Raymond CR. LTP forms 1, 2 and 3: different mechanisms for the "long" in long-term potentiation. Trends Neurosci 2007;30:167.

31. Collingridge GL, Isaac JT, Wang YT. Receptor trafficking and synaptic plasticity. Nat Rev Neurosci 2004;5:952.

32. Malenka RC, Bear MF. LTP and LTD: an embarrassment of riches. Neuron 2004;44:5.

33. Nakazawa K, McHugh TJ, Wilson MA, et al. NMDA receptors, place cells and hippocampal spatial memory. Nat Rev Neurosci 2004;5:361.

34. Bliss TV, Collingridge GL. A synaptic model of memory: long-term potentiation in the hippocampus. Nature 1993;361:31.

35. Lynch MA. Long-term potentiation and memory. Physiol Rev 2004;84:87.

36. Arnsten AF. Catecholamine and second messenger influences on prefrontal cortical networks of "representational knowledge": a rational bridge between genetics and the symptoms of mental illness. Cereb Cortex 2007;17(Suppl 1):i6.

37. Peng S, Zhang Y, Zhang J, et al. ERK in learning and memory: a review of recent research. Int J Mol Sci 2010;11:222.

38. Roberson ED, English JD, Adams JP, et al. The mitogen-activated protein kinase cascade couples PKA and PKC to cAMP response element binding protein phosphorylation in area CA1 of hippocampus. J Neurosci 1999;19:4337.

39. Roberson K, Cameroni I, Toso L, et al. Alterations in phosphorylated cyclic adenosine monophosphate response element of binding protein activity: a pathway for fetal alcohol syndrome-related neurotoxicity. Am J Obstet Gynecol 2009;200:193, e1.

40. Gelinas JN, Banko JL, Peters MM, et al. Activation of exchange protein activated by cyclic-AMP enhances long-lasting synaptic potentiation in the hippocampus. Learn Mem 2008;15:403.

41. Casadio A, Martin KC, Giustetto M, et al. A transient, neuron-wide form of CREB-mediated long-term facilitation can be stabilized at specific synapses by local protein synthesis. Cell 1999;99:221.

42. Bourtchouladze R, Abel T, Berman N, et al. Different training procedures recruit either one or two critical periods for contextual memory consolidation, each of which requires protein synthesis and PKA. Learn Mem 1998;5:365.

43. Chew SJ, Vicario DS, Nottebohm F. Quantal duration of auditory memories. Science 1996;274:1909.

44. Freeman FM, Rose SP, Scholey AB. Two time windows of anisomycin-induced amnesia for passive avoidance training in the day-old chick. Neurobiol Learn Mem 1995;63:291.

45. Grecksch G, Matthies H. Two sensitive periods for the amnesic effect of anisomycin. Pharmacol Biochem Behav 1980;12:663.

46. Bekinschtein P, Cammarota M, Igaz LM, et al. Persistence of long-term memory storage requires a late protein synthesis- and BDNF-dependent phase in the hippocampus. Neuron 2007;53:261.

47. Igaz LM, Vianna MR, Medina JH, et al. Two time periods of hippocampal mRNA synthesis are required for memory consolidation of fear-motivated learning. J Neurosci 2002;22:6781.

48. Rossato JI, Bevilaqua LRM, Izquierdo I, et al. Dopamine controls persistence of long-term memory storage. Science 2009;325:1017.

49. Gvilia I. Underlying brain mechanisms that regulate sleep-wakefulness cycles. Int Rev Neurobiol 2010;93:1.

50. Luppi PH. Neurochemical aspects of sleep regulation with specific focus on slow-wave sleep. World J Biol Psychiatry 2010;11(Suppl 1):4.

51. Frey U, Krug M, Reymann KG, et al. Anisomycin, an inhibitor of protein synthesis, blocks late phases of LTP phenomena in the hippocampal CA1 region in vitro. Brain Res 1988;452:57.

52. Nguyen PV, Abel T, Kandel ER. Requirement of a critical period of transcription for induction of a late phase of LTP. Science 1994;265:1104.

53. Frey U, Morris RG. Synaptic tagging and long-term potentiation. Nature 1997;385:533.

54. Frey U, Morris RG. Weak before strong: dissociating synaptic tagging and plasticity-factor accounts of late-LTP. Neuropharmacology 1998;37:545.

55. Martin KC, Casadio A, Zhu H, et al. Synapse-specific, long-term facilitation of aplysia sensory to motor synapses: a function for local protein synthesis in memory storage. Cell 1997;91:927.

56. Martin KC, Kosik KS. Synaptic tagging – who's it? Nat Rev Neurosci 2002;3:813.

57. Pittenger C, Kandel ER. In search of general mechanisms for long-lasting plasticity: aplysia and the hippocampus. Philos Trans R Soc Lond B Biol Sci 2003;358:757.

58. Huang T, McDonough CB, Abel T. Compartmentalized PKA signaling events are required for synaptic tagging and capture during hippocampal late-phase long-term potentiation. Eur J Cell Biol 2006;85:635.

59. Okada D, Ozawa F, Inokuchi K. Input-specific spine entry of soma-derived Vesl-1S protein conforms to synaptic tagging. Science 2009;324:904.

60. Maret SP, Dorsaz SP, Gurcel L, et al. Homer1a is a core brain molecular correlate of sleep loss. Proc Natl Acad Sci U S A 2007;104:20090.

61. Shema R, Sacktor TC, Dudai Y. Rapid erasure of long-term memory associations in the cortex by an inhibitor of PKM zeta. Science 2007;317:951.

62. Yao Y, Kelly MT, Sajikumar S, et al. PKM zeta maintains late long-term potentiation by N-ethylmaleimide-sensitive factor/GluR2-dependent trafficking of postsynaptic AMPA receptors. J Neurosci 2008;28:7820.

63. Moncada D, Viola H. Induction of long-term memory by exposure to novelty requires protein synthesis: evidence for a behavioral tagging. J Neurosci 2007;27:7476.

64. Walker MP, Stickgold R. Sleep dependent learning and memory consolidation. Neuron 2004;44:121.

65. Gais S, Rasch B, Wagner U, et al. Visual-procedural memory consolidation during sleep blocked by glutamatergic receptor antagonists. J Neurosci 2008;28:5513.

66. Mednick S, Nakayama K, Stickgold R. Sleep-dependent learning: a nap is as good as a night. Nat Neurosci 2003;6:697.

67. Dash PK, Hebert AE, Runyan JD. A unified theory for systems and cellular memory consolidation. Brain Res Brain Res Rev 2004;45:30.

68. Frankland PW, Bontempi B. The organization of recent and remote memories. Nat Rev Neurosci 2005;6:119.

69. Sutherland RJ, Sparks FT, Lehmann H. Hippocampus and retrograde amnesia in the rat model: a modest proposal for the situation of systems consolidation. Neuropsychologia 2010;48(8):2357–69.

70. Rasch B, Born J. Maintaining memories by reactivation. Curr Opin Neurobiol 2007;17:698.

71. Tse D, Langston RF, Kakeyama M, et al. Schemas and memory consolidation. Science 2007;316:76.

72. Wang SH, Morris RG. Hippocampal-neocortical interactions in memory formation, consolidation, and reconsolidation. Annu Rev Psychol 2010;61:49.

73. Nakashiba T, Buhl DL, McHugh TJ, et al. Hippocampal CA3 output is crucial for ripple-associated reactivation and consolidation of memory. Neuron 2009;62:781.

74. Gais S, Albouy G, Boly M, et al. Sleep transforms the cerebral trace of declarative memories. Proc Natl Acad Sci U S A 2007;104:18778.

75. Takashima A, Petersson KM, Rutters F, et al. Declarative memory consolidation in humans: a prospective functional magnetic resonance imaging study. Proc Natl Acad Sci U S A 2006;103:756.

76. Orban P, Rauchs G, Balteau E, et al. Sleep after spatial learning promotes covert reorganization of brain activity. Proc Natl Acad Sci U S A 2006;103:7124.

77. Gordon W. Similarities of recently acquired and re-activated memories in interference. Am J Psychol 1977;90:231.

78. Misanin JR, Miller RR, Lewis DJ. Retrograde amnesia produced by electroconvulsive shock after reactivation of a consolidated memory trace. Science 1968;160:554.

79. Schneider AM, Sherman W. Amnesia: a function of the temporal relation of footshock to electroconvulsive shock. Science 1968;159:219.

80. Lee JL. Memory reconsolidation mediates the strengthening of memories by additional learning. Nat Neurosci 2008;11:1264.

81. Lee JL, Di Ciano P, Thomas KL, et al. Disrupting reconsolidation of drug memories reduces cocaine-seeking behavior. Neuron 2005;47:795.

82. Nader K, Einarsson EO. Memory reconsolidation: an update. Ann N Y Acad Sci 2010;1191:27.

83. Radulovic J, Tronson NC. Molecular specificity of multiple hippocampal processes governing fear extinction. Rev Neurosci 2010;21:1.

84. Mayford M, Bach ME, Huang YY, et al. Control of memory formation through regulated expression of a CaMKII transgene. Science 1996;274:1678.

85. Murchison CF, Zhang XY, Zhang WP, et al. A distinct role for norepinephrine in memory retrieval. Cell 2004;117:131.

86. Barros DM, Izquierdo LA, Mello e Souza T, et al. Molecular signalling pathways in the cerebral cortex are required for retrieval of one-trial avoidance learning in rats. Behav Brain Res 2000;114:183.

87. Izquierdo LA, Barros DM, Ardenghi PG, et al. Different hippocampal molecular requirements for short- and long-term retrieval of one-trial avoidance learning. Behav Brain Res 2000;111:93.

88. Izquierdo LA, Viola H, Barros DM, et al. Novelty enhances retrieval: molecular mechanisms involved in rat hippocampus. Eur J Neurosci 2001;13:1464.

89. Walker MP, Brakefield T, Hobson JA, et al. Dissociable stages of human memory consolidation and reconsolidation. Nature 2003;425:616.

90. Tronson NC, Taylor JR. Molecular mechanisms of memory reconsolidation. Nat Rev Neurosci 2007; 8:262.

91. Stickgold R. Sleep-dependent memory consolidation. Nature 2005;437:1272.

92. Alvarenga TA, Patti CL, Andersen ML, et al. Paradoxical sleep deprivation impairs acquisition, consolidation, and retrieval of a discriminative avoidance task in rats. Neurobiol Learn Mem 2008;90:624.

93. Fischer S, Nitschke MF, Melchert UH, et al. Motor memory consolidation in sleep shapes more effective neuronal representations. J Neurosci 2005;25: 11248.

94. Walker MP, Stickgold R, Alsop D, et al. Sleep-dependent motor memory plasticity in the human brain. Neuroscience 2005;133:911.

95. Diekelmann S, Born J. One memory, two ways to consolidate? Nat Neurosci 2007;10:1085.

96. Aton SJ, Seibt J, Dumoulin M, et al. Mechanisms of sleep-dependent consolidation of cortical plasticity. Neuron 2009;61:454.

97. Frank MG, Issa NP, Stryker MP. Sleep enhances plasticity in the developing visual cortex. Neuron 2001;30:275.

98. Frank MG, Jha SK, Coleman T. Blockade of postsynaptic activity in sleep inhibits developmental plasticity in visual cortex. Neuroreport 2006;17:1459.

99. Kryger M, Roth T, Dement W. Principles and practice of sleep medicine. 4th edition. Philadelphia: Elsevier Saunders; 2000.

100. Rauchs G, Desgranges B, Foret J, et al. The relationships between memory systems and sleep stages. J Sleep Res 2005;14:123.

101. Iber C, Ancoli-Israel S, Chesson A, et al. The AASM manual for the scoring of sleep and associated events: rules, terminology and technical specifications. 1st edition. Westchester (IL): American Academy of Sleep Medicine; 2007.

102. Hobson JA, Pace-Schott EF. The cognitive neuroscience of sleep: neuronal systems, consciousness and learning. Nat Rev Neurosci 2002;3:679.

103. Steriade M, Nunez A, Amzica F. Intracellular analysis of relations between the slow (<1 Hz) neocortical oscillation and other sleep rhythms of the electroencephalogram. J Neurosci 1993; 13:3266.

104. Steriade M. Grouping of brain rhythms in cortico-thalamic systems. Neuroscience 2006;137:1087.

105. Cantero JL, Atienza M, Stickgold R, et al. Sleep-dependent theta oscillations in the human hippocampus and neocortex. J Neurosci 2003;23:10897.

106. Timo-Iaria C, Negrao N, Schmidek WR, et al. Phases and states of sleep in the rat. Physiol Behav 1970;5:1057.

107. Vanderwolf CH. Hippocampal electrical activity and voluntary movement in the rat. Electroencephalogr Clin Neurophysiol 1969;26:407.

108. Axmacher N, Mormann F, Fernandez G, et al. Memory formation by neuronal synchronization. Brain Res Rev 2006;52:170.

109. Buzsaki G. Theta oscillations in the hippocampus. Neuron 2002;33:325.

110. Habib D, Dringenberg HC. Low-frequency-induced synaptic potentiation: a paradigm shift in the field of memory-related plasticity mechanisms? Hippocampus 2010;20:29.

111. Hyman JM, Wyble BP, Goyal V, et al. Stimulation in hippocampal region CA1 in behaving rats yields long-term potentiation when delivered to the peak of theta and long-term depression when delivered to the trough. J Neurosci 2003;23:11725.

112. O'Keefe J, Nadel L. The hippocampus as a cognitive map. Oxford (UK): Oxford University Press; 1978.

113. Aserinsky E, Kleitman N. Regularly occurring periods of eye motility, and concomitant phenomena, during sleep. Science 1953;118:273.

114. Dement W, Kleitman N. Cyclic variations in EEG during sleep and their relation to eye movements, body motility, and dreaming. Electroencephalogr Clin Neurophysiol 1957;9:673.

115. Dement W, Kleitman N. The relation of eye movements during sleep to dream activity: an objective method for the study of dreaming. J Exp Psychol 1957;53:339.

116. Jouvet M, Michel F. [Electromyographic correlations of sleep in the chronic decorticate & mesencephalic cat]. C R Seances Soc Biol Fil 1959;153: 422 [in French].

117. Nishida M, Walker MP. Daytime naps, motor memory consolidation and regionally specific sleep spindles. PLoS One 2007;2:e341.

118. Schabus M, Gruber G, Parapatics S, et al. Sleep spindles and their significance for declarative memory consolidation. Sleep 2004;27:1479.

119. Buzsaki G, Leung LW, Vanderwolf CH. Cellular bases of hippocampal EEG in the behaving rat. Brain Res 1983;287:139.

120. Ylinen A, Bragin A, Nadasdy Z, et al. Sharp wave-associated high-frequency oscillation (200 Hz) in the intact hippocampus: network and intracellular mechanisms. J Neurosci 1995;15:30.

121. De Gennaro L, Ferrara M. Sleep spindles: an overview. Sleep Med Rev 2003;7:423.

122. Isomura Y, Sirota A, Ozen S, et al. Integration and segregation of activity in entorhinal-hippocampal subregions by neocortical slow oscillations. Neuron 2006;52:871.

123. Diekelmann S, Born J. The memory function of sleep. Nat Rev Neurosci 2010;11:114.

124. Hoffman KL, Battaglia FP, Harris K, et al. The upshot of up states in the neocortex: from slow oscillations to memory formation. J Neurosci 2007;27:11838.

125. Eschenko O, Molle M, Born J, et al. Elevated sleep spindle density after learning or after retrieval in rats. J Neurosci 2006;26:12914.

126. Molle M, Yeshenko O, Marshall L, et al. Hippocampal sharp wave-ripples linked to slow oscillations in rat slow-wave sleep. J Neurophysiol 2006; 96:62.

127. Siapas AG, Wilson MA. Coordinated interactions between hippocampal ripples and cortical spindles during slow-wave sleep. Neuron 1998; 21:1123.

128. Sirota A, Csicsvari J, Buhl D, et al. Communication between neocortex and hippocampus during sleep in rodents. Proc Natl Acad Sci U S A 2003;100: 2065.

129. Qin YL, McNaughton BL, Skaggs WE, et al. Memory reprocessing in corticocortical and hippocampocortical neuronal ensembles. Philos Trans R Soc Lond B Biol Sci 1997;352:1525.

130. Steriade M, Timofeev I. Neuronal plasticity in thalamocortical networks during sleep and waking oscillations. Neuron 2003;37:563.

131. Tononi G, Massimini M, Riedner BA. Sleepy dialogues between cortex and hippocampus: who talks to whom? Neuron 2006;52:748.

132. Kudrimoti HS, Barnes CA, McNaughton BL. Reactivation of hippocampal cell assemblies: effects of behavioral state, experience, and EEG dynamics. J Neurosci 1999;19:4090.

133. Cui Z, Wang H, Tan Y, et al. Inducible and reversible NR1 knockout reveals crucial role of the NMDA receptor in preserving remote memories in the brain. Neuron 2004;41:781.

134. Schulz S, Siemer H, Krug M, et al. Direct evidence for biphasic cAMP responsive element-binding protein phosphorylation during long-term potentiation in the rat dentate gyrus in vivo. J Neurosci 1999;19:5683.

135. Trifilieff P, Herry C, Vanhoutte P, et al. Foreground contextual fear memory consolidation requires two independent phases of hippocampal ERK/CREB activation. Learn Mem 2006;13:340.

136. Marshall L, Helgadottir H, Molle M, et al. Boosting slow oscillations during sleep potentiates memory. Nature 2006;444:610.

137. Girardeau G, Benchenane K, Wiener SI, et al. Selective suppression of hippocampal ripples impairs spatial memory. Nat Neurosci 2009;12:1222.

138. Rasch B, Buchel C, Gais S, et al. Odor cues during slow-wave sleep prompt declarative memory consolidation. Science 2007;315:1426.

139. Llinas R, Ribary U. Coherent 40-Hz oscillation characterizes dream state in humans. Proc Natl Acad Sci U S A 1993;90:2078.

140. Steriade M, Contreras D, Amzica F, et al. Synchronization of fast (30–40 Hz) spontaneous oscillations in intrathalamic and thalamocortical networks. J Neurosci 1996;16:2788.

141. Hennevin E, Leconte P. [Study of the relations between paradoxical sleep and learning processes (author's transl)]. Physiol Behav 1977; 18:307 [in French].

142. Peigneux P, Laureys S, Delbeuck X, et al. Sleeping brain, learning brain. The role of sleep for memory systems. Neuroreport 2001;12:A111.

143. Dujardin K, Guerrien A, Leconte P. Sleep, brain activation and cognition. Physiol Behav 1990;47:1271.

144. Stickgold R, James L, Hobson JA. Visual discrimination learning requires sleep after training. Nat Neurosci 2000;3:1237.

145. Hipolide DC, Tufik S, Raymond R, et al. Heterogeneous effects of rapid eye movement sleep deprivation on binding to alpha- and beta-adrenergic receptor subtypes in rat brain. Neuroscience 1998;86:977.

146. Vassalli A, Dijk DJ. Sleep function: current questions and new approaches. Eur J Neurosci 2009; 29:1830.

147. Hellman K, Abel T. Fear conditioning increases NREM sleep. Behav Neurosci 2007;121:310.

148. Hanlon EC, Faraguna U, Vyazovskiy VV, et al. Effects of skilled training on sleep slow wave activity and cortical gene expression in the rat. Sleep 2009;32:719.

149. Huber R, Ghilardi MF, Massimini M, et al. Arm immobilization causes cortical plastic changes and locally decreases sleep slow wave activity. Nat Neurosci 2006;9(9):1169–76.

150. Huber R, Ghilardi MF, Massimini M, et al. Local sleep and learning. Nature 2004;430:78.

151. Szymusiak R. Hypothalamic versus neocortical control of sleep. Curr Opin Pulm Med 2010;16:530.

152. Walker MP, Brakefield T, Seidman J, et al. Sleep and the time course of motor skill learning. Learn Mem 2003;10:275.

153. Drosopoulos S, Windau E, Wagner U, et al. Sleep enforces the temporal order in memory. PLoS One 2007;2:e376.

154. Kuriyama K, Stickgold R, Walker MP. Sleep-dependent learning and motor-skill complexity. Learn Mem 2004;11:705.

155. Steenland H, Wu V, Fukushima H, et al. CaMKIV over-expression boosts cortical 4-7 Hz oscillations during learning and 1-4 Hz delta oscillations during sleep. Mol Brain 2010;3:16.

156. Borbely A, Achermann P. The human circadian timing system and sleep-wake regulation. In: Kryger M, Roth T, Dement W, editors. Principles and practice of sleep medicine. Philadelphia: WB Saunders; 2000. p. 377.

157. Gerstner JR, Lyons LC, Wright KP Jr, et al. Cycling behavior and memory formation. J Neurosci 2009; 29:12824.

158. Takahashi JS, Hong HK, Ko CH, et al. The genetics of mammalian circadian order and disorder: implications for physiology and disease. Nat Rev Genet 2008;9:764.

159. Cirelli C, Tononi G. Differential expression of plasticity-related genes in waking and sleep and their regulation by the noradrenergic system. J Neurosci 2000;20:9187.

160. Dolci C, Montaruli A, Roveda E, et al. Circadian variations in expression of the trkB receptor in adult rat hippocampus. Brain Res 2003;994:67.

161. Duffield GE, Best JD, Meurers BH, et al. Circadian programs of transcriptional activation, signaling, and protein turnover revealed by microarray analysis of mammalian cells. Curr Biol 2002;12:551.

162. Lowrey PL, Takahashi JS. Mammalian circadian biology: elucidating genome-wide levels of temporal organization. Annu Rev Genomics Hum Genet 2004;5:407.

163. Panda S, Antoch MP, Miller BH, et al. Coordinated transcription of key pathways in the mouse by the circadian clock. Cell 2002;109:307.

164. Eckel-Mahan KL, Storm DR. Circadian rhythms and memory: not so simple as cogs and gears. EMBO Rep 2009;10:584.

165. Hendricks JC, Sehgal A, Pack AI. The need for a simple animal model to understand sleep. Prog Neurobiol 2000;61:339.

166. Fischer S, Hallschmid M, Elsner AL, et al. Sleep forms memory for finger skills. Proc Natl Acad Sci U S A 2002;99:11987.

167. Korman M, Doyon J, Doljansky J, et al. Daytime sleep condenses the time course of motor memory consolidation. Nat Neurosci 2007;10:1206.

168. Stickgold R, Whidbee D, Schirmer B, et al. Visual discrimination task improvement: a multi-step process occurring during sleep. J Cogn Neurosci 2000;12:246.

169. Foster DJ, Wilson MA. Reverse replay of behavioural sequences in hippocampal place cells during the awake state. Nature 2006;440:680.

170. Kali S, Dayan P. Off-line replay maintains declarative memories in a model of hippocampal-neocortical interactions. Nat Neurosci 2004;7:286.

171. Pavlides C, Winson J. Influences of hippocampal place cell firing in the awake state on the activity of these cells during subsequent sleep episodes. J Neurosci 1989;9:2907.

172. Skaggs WE, McNaughton BL. Replay of neuronal firing sequences in rat hippocampus during sleep following spatial experience. Science 1996;271: 1870.

173. Ganguly-Fitzgerald I, Donlea J, Shaw PJ. Waking experience affects sleep need in Drosophila. Science 2006;313:1775.

174. Hellman K, Hernandez P, Park A, et al. Genetic evidence for a role for protein kinase A in the maintenance of sleep and thalamocortical oscillations. Sleep 2010;33:19.

175. Gottlieb DJ, O'Connor GT, Wilk JB. Genome-wide association of sleep and circadian phenotypes. BMC Med Genet 2007;8(Suppl 1):S9.

176. Hendricks JC, Finn SM, Panckeri KA, et al. Rest in Drosophila is a sleep-like state. Neuron 2000;25:129.

177. Joiner WJ, Crocker A, White BH, et al. Sleep in Drosophila is regulated by adult mushroom bodies. Nature 2006;441:757.

178. Wu MN, Ho K, Crocker A, et al. The effects of caffeine on sleep in Drosophila require PKA activity, but not the adenosine receptor. J Neurosci 2009;29:11029.

179. Crocker A, Sehgal A. Genetic analysis of sleep. Genes Dev 2010;24:1220.

180. Isiegas C, McDonough C, Huang T, et al. A novel conditional genetic system reveals that increasing neuronal cAMP enhances memory and retrieval. J Neurosci 2008;28(24):6220–30.

181. Cardin JA, Carlen M, Meletis K, et al. Targeted optogenetic stimulation and recording of neurons in vivo using cell-type-specific expression of Channelrhodopsin-2. Nat Protoc 2010;5:247.

Brain Stimulation During Sleep

Lisa Marshall, PhD[a,*], Jan Born, PhD[a,b]

KEYWORDS

- Transcranial direct current stimulation
- Transcranial magnetic stimulation • Electroencephalogram
- Slow oscillation • Non–rapid eye movement sleep
- Memory

Previous articles have reviewed the memory function of sleep in humans and animals. This article deals essentially with cortical polarization and the induction of brain rhythms during sleep via electric and magnetic stimulations of the brain and the resultant functional relevance. Although sensory stimulation as used in evoked potential studies to measure information processing during sleep also presents a means to stimulate brain activity, the authors do not deal with this literature in this article, but the readers are referred for this literature to several comprehensive articles.[1,2]

HISTORICAL PERSPECTIVE AND STIMULATION PROTOCOLS

According to a thorough historical account on brain polarization by Priori,[3] beneficial effects of a direct electric current delivered to the scalp of a patient with migraine was first reported already in the sixteenth century. The generator of this current was then a live torpedo fish. Since then, effects of galvanic currents on patients with mental disorders, used as a stimulating or sedative treatment, have been observed. These studies, using mostly direct current (DC) stimulation, revealed some consistent results, such as the induction of opposite effects when reversing stimulation polarities of the DC current. However, overall results remained rather mixed, and this together with the strong advancement in neuropsychopharmacology led to a progressive abandonment of DC stimulation in clinical use and a strong reduction in research.

Electrosleep and electroanesthesia involve a combination of pulsed and direct currents or interrupted DCs. Although electrosleep and electroanesthesia are often used synonymously, electroanesthesia, which aims to induce unconsciousness for conducting painless human surgery, uses stronger currents and is often associated with undesirable side effects.[4] The electrosleep procedure was used mostly in the Soviet Union at the beginning of the twentieth century for the treatment of various ailments, such as anxiety, insomnia, pain, and depression.[5,6] In the United States, the terms cranial electrotherapy stimulation, cerebral electrotherapy, and transcerebral electrotherapy are used rather than electrosleep.[7] Current is usually applied in an anterior-posterior direction, using electrodes bilaterally placed over the eyes or frontal poles and over the occipital, mastoid, or neck regions. The polarity of anterior electrodes in relation to the posterior electrodes is less consistent across studies.[4,8] Stimulation usually uses rectangular pulses of about 1 millisecond duration (typically 0.4–2.0 millisecond), reoccurring at a frequency between 2 Hz and 200 Hz, with current strengths in the range of 0.03 mA to a few milliamperes. But currents up to 20 mA have also been reported. In addition, DC bias currents have been inconsistently used. For therapy, daily stimulation sessions in the range of 20 minutes to 1 hour and more have been reported, given for up to 20 sessions.[4,5]

This work was supported by the DFG (SFB 654).
a Department of Neuroendocrinology, Building 50.1, University of Lübeck, Ratzeburger Allee 160, 23538 Lübeck, Germany
b Institute of Pyschology and Behavioral Neurobiology, University of Tübingen, Tübingen, Germany
* Corresponding author.
E-mail address: marshall@uni-luebeck.de

Sleep Med Clin 6 (2011) 85–95
doi:10.1016/j.jsmc.2010.12.003

Transcerebral electrotherapy typically takes place in a darkened and quiet room but during wakefulness. Nevertheless, nocturnal electrotherapy has been recommended for treating insomnia, and beneficial effects on sleep occurring after the acute treatment have been indicated; yet the double-blind nature of the studies is limited because of subjects feeling the stimulation.[4,6]

At present, there is a greater transparency in the modes of brain electric stimulation, although different terminologies are in part still circulating. Present day terms pertain less to the investigated function but rather to the mode of electric stimulation. The site of electrode application, polarity, stimulation duration, and electrode size are further details that can deviate strongly between studies dependent on experimental question.[9] Transcranial DC stimulation (tDCS) refers to the application of a steady current throughout the stimulation period. A variation of this current is intermittent tDCS, in which during the stimulation period intervals of tDCS alternate with periods devoid of stimulation. This procedure was specifically used to extend the total time of stimulation across a complete period of pronounced slow wave sleep (SWS) extending for more than 30 minutes while limiting electric charge[10] (SI unit of electric charge, coulomb; 1 coulomb is the amount of electric charge transported in 1 second by a steady current of 1 A). Although the application of weak electric currents, as used in present day protocols, is regarded as safe, there are still no universal safety guidelines.[11-13] However, undesirable side effects are rarely reported. Of more than 90 subjects receiving weak electric current stimulation in the authors' studies only 1 subject, who also revealed quite asymmetric 10:20 head size measurements, reported a sustained headache. Transcranial alternating current stimulation (tACS) refers to AC stimulation fluctuating around zero potential, and a further mode combines alternating current stimulation with a DC bias, for example, slow oscillation tDCS[14] for which details are given later.

In addition to electric brain stimulation, transcranial magnetic stimulation (TMS) is being increasingly used to selectively enhance or suppress, as by virtual reversible lesions, neuronal activity. TMS can be delivered as single pulses, as double (paired) pulses, as rapid sequences of pulses at rates of up to 100 Hz (repetitive TMS), or in patterns (eg, TMS theta bursts). Cortical and corticospinal responses are decisively dependent on temporal factors, for example, paired pulses with short (eg, <7 millisecond) or long interstimulus intervals induce either intracortical inhibition or facilitation, respectively. Similarly, the frequency of repetitive TMS determines whether inhibition or excitation predominates in the stimulated area, with most evidence pointing toward underlying long-term potentiation– and long-term depression–like synaptic mechanisms.[15-18]

The first important difference in TMS and electric brain stimulation is the relatively stronger focal nature of the applied magnetic field and therefore of the induced electric field during TMS as compared with the more widespread electric field produced within the brain after application of weak electric currents to the scalp, although the precise stimulation techniques can prove to be decisive.[19-21] Secondly, owing to the different physical properties, both types of stimulation differ in the primary nature of interaction with brain tissue. The sharp focus of the magnetic field together with the brief pulses in which TMS is delivered leads primarily to suprathreshold modulations presumably on cortical axons and direct changes in neuronal firing rates. By contrast, the effects of stimulation using weak electric currents on spontaneous neuronal activity are attributed to the degree in which transmembrane potentials are more subtly shifted in the depolarizing or hyperpolarizing direction.[22-24]

STIMULATING THE BRAIN DURING SWS

An important common general feature of brain electric and magnetic stimulations is the dependence of effects on brain state, which is applicable for sleep versus wakefulness as well as for different sleep stages and modes of wakefulness (eg, quiet vs active wakefulness). In wakefulness, the dependence on ongoing oscillatory electroencephalogram (EEG) activity underlying specific cognitive functions has been investigated in particular using tACS and patterned TMS.[25] During sleep, a main focus of the brain stimulation has been the slow oscillation rhythm dominant during non–rapid eye movement (NREM) sleep and distinctly increasing at the transition into SWS.[26-28]

The reason for the strong focus on SWS is the underlying EEG slow sleep oscillation of around 1 Hz (approximately 0.75 Hz in humans and approximately 1.5 Hz in rats), that is, a prominent oscillating electric field potential that hallmarks this sleep stage. This macroscopic field potential is well defined at the cellular level. Intracellular recordings of cortical cells reveal an alternation of the membrane potential between a depolarized (up) state with neuronal firing and a hyperpolarized (down) state.[29] Correspondingly, the local field potential and EEG reflect an alteration between increased wakelike neuronal firing (up-state) and global neuronal silence with the up-states expressed as surface-positive and down-states as surface-negative EEG waves.[30–32] The slow oscillation is generated within neocortical networks, whereby a grouping influence of the slow oscillation on thalamocortical spindles has been established such that periods of cortical hyperpolarization are followed by strong rebound spindle activity.[32–34] The underlying concept regarding the functional significance of the slow oscillation is that presumably through neocortical efferent pathways, the activity of other brain regions can synchronize with the neocortical slow oscillation, for instance, the thalamically generated spindles, the sharp-wave ripple activity of the hippocampus, as well as the activity of the brainstem noradrenergic neurons in the locus coeruleus and the cholinergic neurons of the pedunculopontine nucleus, structures that all appear not to independently generate sleep slow oscillations.[35–39] Thus, depending on the excitability level of the neocortex, that is, being in the up- or down-state, subcortical afferent and corticocortical activity is either suppressed or highly efficient.[40–42] In sleep, the emergence of the slow oscillation itself is associated with even slower endogenous NREM–rapid eye movement (REM) sleep–associated shifts in transcortical potential level exhibiting a steep surface-negative cortical DC potential shift at the transition into SWS and a steep positive shift at the transition into REM sleep, the sources of which are still to be determined.[43,44]

The application of both rhythmic electric and magnetic stimulation (at approximately 0.75 Hz and 0.8 Hz, respectively) at the transition into and during SWS is associated with an enhancement of slow oscillatory as well as sleep spindle activity as depicted in **Fig. 1**A.[26,27] Intermittent tDCS over a 30-minute period consisting of alternating 30-second epochs of anodal current at +260 µA and zero current slightly enhanced slow wave activity up to 4 Hz (SWA).[10] A most pronounced widespread enhancement in slow oscillation activity was found with rhythmic tDCS oscillating at a frequency of the human slow oscillation (ie, 0.75 Hz) between zero and +260 µA, applied bilaterally via prefrontolateral electrode sites relative to mastoid references.[14,26] The increase in slow oscillatory EEG power was measured during the five 1-minute intervals immediately succeeding the five 5-minute epochs of continuous slow oscillation tDCS. Enhancement was most pronounced for the slow oscillation band (0.5–1.0 Hz) across anterior to posterior locations. Power within the neighboring SWA frequency band (1–4 Hz) only tended to increase. Slow oscillation stimulation simultaneously enhanced EEG power within the frequency range of the slow frontal spindles (8–12 Hz,

at the frontal midline site) as well as slow spindle counts during the 1-minute stimulation-free intervals. For up to 5 seconds after termination of slow oscillation stimulation, ongoing EEG activity was transiently entrained to the stimulating slow oscillation current.[26] Because the amplitude of the slow oscillation tDCS produced potential fields in the cortical tissue of a size similar to those observed during endogenously generated sleep slow oscillations, these results suggest that slow oscillation field fluctuations are a naturally efficient signal for enhancing synchronized network activity of the neocortex.[42,45]

It is to note that sleep spindles as the hallmark of stage 2 sleep typically reveal in this sleep stage frequencies that are typically centered on approximately 12.5 Hz and approximately 14. 5 Hz at the frontal and centroparietal sites, respectively.[46] However, during deep NREM sleep, particularly evident during stage 4 sleep, slow spindle frequencies can range down to 9 Hz with frequencies centered at approxiamtely10 Hz[47]; Fig. 3 supporting information of Mölle and colleagues.[48]

The assessment of single TMS pulses applied at about the frequency of the endogenous slow oscillation at 0.8 Hz for approximately 50-second blocks increased both the slow oscillation during the 50-second TMS-on intervals as well as SWA (0.25–4 Hz) in the 1-minute TMS-off intervals.[27] Furthermore, the positive portion of the TMS-evoked wave was associated with a significant increase in spindle (12–15 Hz) amplitude. The amplitude of the induced individual slow oscillations was dependent on stimulation site with maximal responses occurring over the sensorimotor cortex. However, it is to note that stimulation over the orbitofrontal cortex, a hot spot for slow oscillation generation, in that study was not probed by TMS for technical reasons. The negative peak of TMS-induced slow waves also showed a topographic delay gradient similar to the traveling wave property of the endogenous slow oscillation.

Electric and magnetic slow oscillation stimulation procedures reveal strong dependence on the brain state. Unlike during NREM sleep, TMS pulses delivered rhythmically at a rate of 1 Hz during wakefulness did not evoke slow oscillations but were associated with long-range, spatially and temporally differentiated responses (within the 400-millisecond poststimulation interval). Electric slow oscillation tDCS was also less efficient during wakefulness than NREM sleep, inducing only a local increase in slow oscillation EEG power close to the frontal stimulation sites. EEG activity in the spindle frequency range was not affected by transcranial brain stimulation (electric or

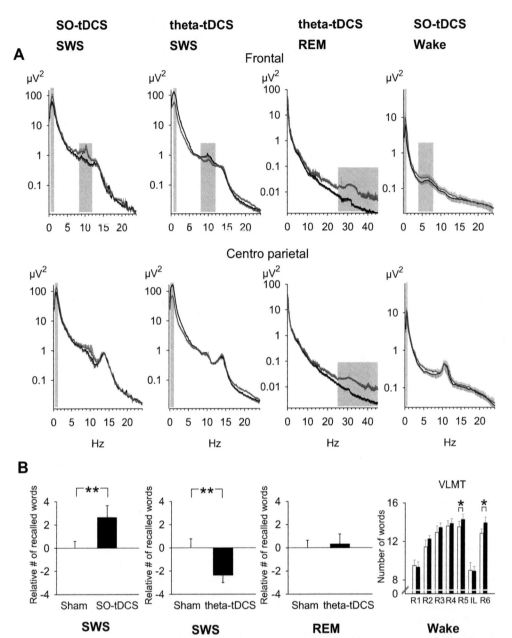

Fig. 1. Effect of oscillating tDCS on endogenous EEG activity and on learning and memory, depending on the oscillation frequency of stimulation and on brain state. (*A*) Comparative changes in the EEG spectral power within 1-minute intervals after termination of 0.75-Hz slow oscillation (SO) tDCS and 5-Hz theta tDCS during SWS, REM, and wakefulness at frontal (*top*) and centroparietal (*bottom*) recording sites (curves: red, stimulation; black, sham). Gray areas indicate frequency bands significantly modified by stimulation. (*B*) Effects of stimulation on retention of word paired-associates in declarative learning tasks and on encoding of memories during the Verbal Learning and Memory Test (VLMT). Stimulation during SWS at the 0.75-Hz SO tDCS frequency increases SO and slow frontal spindle activity together with an enhancing effect on declarative memory retention, whereas the opposite effects on EEG and memory performance are produced when tDCS during SWS is applied at the 5-Hz theta frequency. During REM sleep, theta tDCS enhances gamma (25–45 Hz) activity with no effect on memory retention. The relative number of recalled words during sham is normalized to zero. During wakefulness, SO tDCS enhances theta activity, aside from a local increase in SO activity, and this effect was accompanied by improved encoding performance. The number of words recalled on the fifth presentation of a standard word list (R5) and on free recall (R6) immediately succeeding presentation of an interference list (IL) were enhanced compared with sham (bars: black, tDCS; open, sham). *$P<.05$; **$P<.01$.

magnetic) at the slow oscillation frequency during wakefulness.[27,49] However, slow oscillation tDCS over prefrontal sites during wakefulness induced a widespread enhancement in EEG theta power. It was observed that tDCS oscillating at 5-Hz theta frequency (theta tDCS) suppressed endogenous slow oscillation activity (0.5–1.0 Hz) and frontal slow spindle activity (8–12 Hz) when applied during early NREM and SWS.[26] The theta tDCS–induced suppression of slow oscillation activity during NREM sleep together with the robust increase in endogenous theta activity after slow oscillation tDCS observed in the wake state indicate a preferred coupling between potential field rhythms at the 2 frequencies, that is, the approximately 0.75-Hz slow oscillation and approximately 5-Hz theta frequency, that may reflect a basic functional relationship between the cortical networks underlying these oscillations. Spontaneous EEG slow oscillation activity emerges on a global scale during SWS, whereas theta activity prevails in the active waking state. In fact, based on the positive correlation between EEG theta activity in waking and SWA during subsequent sleep, it has been proposed that both oscillations are markers of a common homeostatic sleep process relating sleep depth to the amount of information encoded during prior waking.[50–52] Application of the same 5-Hz theta tDCS which suppressed slow oscillatory activity, during NREM sleep induced EEG gamma band activity during REM sleep (25–45 Hz; L.M., unpublished observations, 2010; see **Fig. 1**A). This induction presents a further example of field potential fluctuations of one rhythm affecting network activity of a presumed functionally related brain rhythm (see **Fig. 1**).

A stimulation procedure similar to that used for 1-Hz TMS in humans by Massimini and colleagues[27] was applied in rats by Vyazovskiy and colleagues[28] using intracortical electric stimulation with monophasic square pulses delivered in most experiments at a slow rate of 0.2 Hz during NREM sleep. As in the earlier-mentioned human study, the stimulation evoked slow waves that were temporally associated with sleep spindles (approximately 15 Hz). Because individual waves were determined within the wider frequency band of 0.5 to 4.0 Hz, the term slow waves and not slow oscillation is used in this study. The amplitude of the evoked slow wave was generally dependent on the background activity during the 2-second interval preceding the stimulation, that is, it was diminished for high-amplitude background activity and conversely enhanced for low-amplitude background activity during this interval. Furthermore, the reduction in amplitude of the evoked slow wave was greater the shorter the latency of the evoked slow wave to the preceding spontaneous high amplitude slow oscillation. Note, minimum amplitudes for evoked slow waves were obtained within a 200 ms interval following the peak of an endogenous slow wave (ie, when triggered close to the down-to-up-state transition). Of importance is that for spontaneous slow waves a similar short-lasting refractory period following large amplitude slow waves, defined as larger than the median slow wave amplitude, was found.[28] A different temporal relationship was revealed, however, for trains of several succeeding spontaneous slow oscillations examined in humans. In fact here, peak-to-peak amplitudes were highest for "middle" slow oscillations that were preceded and followed by other slow oscillations, whereas "initial" slow oscillations that were followed but not preceded by another slow oscillation exhibited a significantly smaller amplitude and were similar in amplitude to "final" slow oscillations terminating a train of spontaneously occurring oscillations (Matthias Mölle, PhD, Lübeck, Germany, personal communication, 2010). The putative intracellular and/or extracellular substances and associated network activity that specifically underlie this kind of waxing and waning in cortical slow oscillations sequences is as yet completely obscure.[53–55]

TMS STIMULATION TO PROBE BRAIN EXCITABILITY DURING SLEEP

TMS has been used to assess excitability of motor cortical areas as well as responsiveness of corticospinal pathways during sleep. Basically, TMS generates an electric current across the scalp and skull and in brain tissue via electromagnetic induction. Fields produced by TMS preferentially depolarize and subsequently discharge action potentials of axons running in the plane tangential to the curvature of the head because axons are depolarized most efficiently by electric fields oriented in the plane parallel to their path.[56] A suprathreshold TMS pulse given, for example, to the primary motor cortex, evokes multiple descending volleys in corticospinal neurons, which then drive spinal motor neurons to discharge. Amplitude, latency, and form of the resultant motor evoked potential measured at a peripheral muscle reflect excitation of the corticospinal system. Many details of the TMS effect on this pathway are, however, still unclear.[57] Paired-pulse TMS using a subthreshold conditioning stimulus (S1) followed by a suprathreshold test pulse (S2) during different sleep states has been used to investigate comparative differences in motor cortical (as opposed to corticospinal) activity. Effects of S1 on the motor evoked potential on S2 is assumed to reflect essentially short-interval intracortical inhibition (SICI) if the interstimulus intervals lie between 1 and 6 milliseconds or intracortical facilitation (ICF) for interstimulus intervals of 8 to 30 milliseconds. Different neuronal circuitries are presumed to be involved in producing SICI and ICF as inferred from findings revealing (1) different thresholds for induction and (2) discrepant sensitivity to induced current flow direction as well as to neuropharmacologic manipulations.[58–60]

Several studies using single-pulse TMS during sleep suggested that corticospinal excitability is generally reduced during sleep as compared with wakefulness.[61–63] However, differences between sleep stages using single-pulse TMS indicated significantly higher corticospinal excitability in SWS than in stage 2 sleep.[62,63] On the other hand, paired-pulse TMS revealed stronger SICI for deep NREM sleep, including stage 2 to stage 3 transitions than for wakefulness, whereas SICI in REM sleep and light NREM sleep stage 2 did not differ from wakefulness. ICF during deep as well as light NREM sleep did not differ significantly from wakefulness, and in REM sleep, ICF was absent.[64] For SWS, SICI seems to be increased and intracortical facilitation maintained at the level of wakefulness. In an exploratory study, patients with epilepsy revealed significantly reduced and absent SICI during NREM sleep as compared with healthy subjects,[65] which coincides with their increased seizure probability during sleep and underscores the relevance of increased SICI during NREM sleep for normal function.

Motor cortical excitability was also assessed by paired-pulse stimulation during the approximate 5-minute period on awakening from sleep assumed to be an interval still reflecting corticospinal excitability during the previous sleep state.[66] This assumption is essentially derived from the measurements of brain metabolic activity using $H_2^{15}O$ positron emission tomography in which reestablishment of waking regional brain activity patterns in anterior cortical regions were not established until approximately 20 minutes after awakening.[67] The main finding was increased ICF after awakening from REM sleep than after SWS awakening or for stimulation during presleep wakefulness, which contrasts with the earlier-mentioned findings on REM sleep by Salih and colleagues[64] applying paired-pulse TMS during REM sleep. For all these studies applying paired-pulse TMS during or after sleep, it must be kept in mind that the primary outcome measure, that is, the motor evoked potential, like for single pulse TMS, is recorded from a peripheral muscle. This

measure principally questions whether effects reflect intracortical inhibition or facilitation that is uncontaminated by spinal or subcortical mechanisms.[63]

In getting closer to the neurophysiology of the slow oscillation rhythm of SWS, Bergmann and colleagues[68] measured the TMS-induced motor evoked potential time locked to online-detected slow oscillation up- and down-states in SWS. Although motor evoked potentials were generally reduced during NREM sleep compared with wakefulness, motor responses were consistently higher during up-states than during down-states of the slow oscillation. In contrast, during wakefulness, corticospinal excitability to single-pulse TMS during different phases of a slow oscillation potential that was produced by slow oscillation tDCS over the motor cortex did not differ.[69] These findings underline the fact that applied weak electric currents such as slow oscillation tDCS do not seem to impose electric oscillations on the cortical neuronal membrane potential independent of the spontaneous network activity. Furthermore, the differential evoked TMS response during the different phases of the slow oscillation indicates that the efficiency of stimulation is also strongly dependent on endogenous substate fluctuations during SWS. Such differences in response to electric or magnetic stimulation on substate activity may also underlie the earlier-described difference found for ICF during REM sleep and on awakening from REM sleep as described by De Gennaro and colleagues[66] and Salih and colleagues.[64]

BRAIN STIMULATION DURING SLEEP, MEMORY, AND HOMEOSTATIC REGULATION

The induction of oscillatory activity in the brain is a promising first step toward noninvasively investigating the function of brain electric rhythms. In particular for the sleep slow oscillation, electric and magnetic, and also sensory, stimulations[70,71] have proven efficient in enhancing and also in specifically suppressing ongoing brain rhythms. In this section, the authors describe functional implications resulting from induced brain rhythms. As already mentioned, the effect of brain stimulation on EEG activity is determined strongly by the present brain state[26,27,49] and so also is its effect on memory consolidation. The effect on memory consolidation has been studied as one major function of sleep that is essentially regulated by ongoing brain electric activity.

Basically, studies investigating the effect on sleep-dependent memory consolidation have been guided by a dual process view on memory consolidation underscoring the differential benefit for memory from the 2 core sleep stages, that is, in humans SWS and REM sleep. Using a so-called split night experimental design results have shown that the SWS-rich sleep of the first half of the night as compared with wakefulness and the REM-rich sleep of the late night is particularly beneficial for the consolidation of hippocampus-dependent declarative memories (word paired-associates, stories, visuospatial memories) in humans, whereas the retention of procedural memories for perceptual and motor skills as well as emotional memories were found to benefit more from REM-rich sleep in the late-night half.[72–74] Regarding the neurophysiologic bases for the consolidation of declarative memories, an underlying dialog between the hippocampus and neocortex is assumed, whereby the neocortical sleep slow oscillation groups hippocampal sharp-wave ripple events, accompanying the replay of freshly encoded memories in hippocampal networks, in parallel to thalamocortical spindle activity.[34,38,39,75,76] The parallel promotion of sharp wave–ripples and spindles facilitates the formation of so-called spindle-ripple events that have been considered a mechanism whereby hippocampal memory information is transferred to the neocortex for long-term storage.[34,39,44] Although the relevance of the strong depolarization associated with sharp wave–ripples events for the hippocampal to neocortical information transfer was proposed over 20 years ago,[77,78] a consistent hippocampoprefrontal spike-timing relationships driven by hippocampal sharp wave/ripple events during SWS as well as a causal involvement of sharp wave–ripples in the consolidation of memory could only recently be experimentally demonstrated.[79,80]

On this background, the first studies using brain stimulation during sleep to investigate sleep-dependent consolidation of declarative memories applied the weak electric current prefrontally during a period of early SWS-rich sleep, specifically at the transition into SWS.[10,26] In one of these studies, slow oscillation tDCS over prefrontal cortex during early SWS-rich sleep resulted in a strong topographically widespread increase in endogenous slow oscillation and slow frontal spindle activity, together with a robust improvement in the retention of verbal and nonverbal paired-associates, whereas memory performance on procedural tasks (mirror tracing skill, finger sequence tapping) was not significantly affected (verbal paired-associates, see **Fig. 1**B).[26] In patients with schizophrenia, slow oscillation stimulation during SWS similarly was effective in enhancing retention of declarative memories (Robert Göder, MD, Kiel, Germany, personal

communication, 2010). Together, the common increment in retention of declarative memories, slow oscillation, and associated slow spindle activity strongly suggests that the endogenous slow oscillation during SWS has a causal role in memory consolidation. The specificity of this effect was underscored by control experiments in which 25 minutes of slow oscillation tDCS delivered shortly before awakening, that is, at the REM-rich end of the nocturnal period of retention sleep, remained without effect on retention performance. Effects of stimulation on retrieval operations from long-term memory, working memory operations, or mood during the time of postsleep retrieval testing could also be excluded as confounding factors on memory performance. Improved mood was revealed after a shorter 3-hour period of retention sleep in a second study when applying intermittent tDCS over a 30-minute period consisting of alternating 15-second epochs of anodal current at +260 μA and no current.[10] Intermittent tDCS produced a significant improvement in the retention of declarative memories for word pairs the subjects had learned before the nocturnal stimulation period. In addition, the 15-second stimulation-on as compared with current-off epochs revealed an enhancement in EEG slow oscillatory activity (<2 Hz). One elegant study using mild acoustic stimuli to suppress SWA (0.5–4 Hz) throughout the night in elderly individuals without significantly altering sleep stages as scored by Rechtschaffen and Kales[81] indicated a further function of slow oscillatory activity. The significant reduction in SWA impaired encoding of pictures learned after suppression of SWA. Thus, slow oscillatory EEG activity seems relevant for subsequent encoding related to hippocampal activation as measured in this study by the degree of subsequent success in retrieving the learnt materials.[71]

The absence of memory enhancement when slow oscillation tDCS induced only a local enhancement in slow oscillatory activity during wakefulness[49] underscores the functional relevance of widespread cortical slow oscillatory field fluctuations for memory consolidation and also suggests the involvement of additional neuromodulatory mechanisms that are present specifically during the state of SWS. Moreover, the application of 5-Hz theta tDCS at the transition into SWS counteracted effects of slow oscillation tDCS on both endogenous EEG power and memory performance, the decrease in slow oscillatory and frontal slow spindle activity within the 1-minute intervals succeeding stimulation periods coincided with a decrement in retention of word paired-associates supportive of a causal link between slow oscillatory and spindle EEG activity and sleep-dependent consolidation of declarative memories (L.M., unpublished observations, 2010). Results furthermore indicate the functional relevance for consolidation of the timing of these endogenous rhythms in relation to sleep onset and/or sleep cycle because in the study, memory retention was impaired after theta tDCS at SWS onset despite a subsequent strong rebound in sleep slow oscillation and slow spindle power within the 30-minute interval following cessation of theta tDCS. Moreover, although this rebound activity was not sufficient in terms of memory consolidation, results nevertheless indicate the involvement of a homeostatically regulated mechanism as a response to stimulation. Various biochemical, hemodynamic, and related metabolic processes occur as a consequence of tDCS.[82–85] However, to what extent the homeostatic mechanism of the neuronal networks underlying slow oscillatory and slow spindle activity depend on such processes remains to be determined.

In a study by the authors, also briefly mentioned earlier, in which 5-Hz theta tDCS was applied during REM sleep in the second half of the night, stimulation led to enhanced widespread activity in the gamma frequency range (L.M., unpublished observations, 2010; **Fig. 1**). However, despite this distinct increase in gamma activity, an EEG rhythm thought to transiently link cell assemblies processing closely related information,[86] retention of neither declarative paired-associates nor procedural tasks was affected by stimulation. This result may be considered as consistent with the sequential hypothesis proposed originally by Giuditta and colleagues[87] assuming that REM sleep facilitates memory consolidation only together with preceding memory processing during SWS.[88,89] However, the role of REM sleep and associated oscillatory EEG activity for memory processing is presently obscure.

SLEEP AFTER TMS-INDUCED PLASTICITY

Rather than presleep learning protocols, several studies used specific presleep TMS protocols to induce cortical plasticity and to study the effects of sleep on the plastic mechanisms presumed to underlie memory formation.[90–92] Although stimulation was not applied during sleep, all of these studies revealed location-specific correlation between the induced cortical plasticity and intensity of subsequent sleep in terms of slow oscillatory power. In these studies during wakefulness before sleep, median nerve stimulation was followed by a TMS pulse at intervals leading either to a synaptic long-term potentiation or a depression-like activity in the motor cortex, as measured by motor evoked potentials. These local changes in plasticity in the evening before sleep resulted in modulation of slow oscillatory activity, slow spindle activity, and also frontal theta activity during NREM sleep. The modulations in slow wave and slow spindle activity were hereby correlated to the size of the effect of the paired associative stimulation on the motor evoked potential measured before sleep.[90,92] The modulations in ongoing EEG activity during SWS occurring not only in the motor and sensorimotor cortical regions but also at focal prefrontal areas suggest a spread of neuronal excitation via corticocortical connections. Taken together, these studies support both the concept of activity-dependent local sleep regulation, whereby induced plasticity during waking predicts enhanced SWA during following SWS as well as the role of sleep in memory consolidation. In support of this finding is the finding that changes in motor cortical excitability induced by paired associative stimulation in the evening were maintained across the night of sleep but disappeared when subjects remained awake.[90]

SUMMARY

Brain stimulation during sleep by weak electric currents or magnetic pulses represents an effective tool for the investigation of characteristic brain EEG rhythms and their interactions during sleep as well as of the roles these rhythms play for cortical plasticity and memory consolidation. Together, the studies discussed here consistently underscore the strong dependence of induced EEG rhythms and their functional effects on the ongoing brain activity. In a more general sense, inasmuch as the applied weak electric currents mimic endogenous cortical field potential oscillations, theses studies lend strong support to the reemerging concept that endogenous fields are per se of physiologic and functional significance.[93] The application of weak electric currents therefore presents a promising approach for investigating the function of brain rhythms in behavior as well as within cortical networks.

ACKNOWLEDGMENTS

We would like to acknowledge Dr Matthias Mölle for his comments on this article. Furthermore, we greatly acknowledge the student movement "Lübeck Fights for Its University" in the ongoing struggle against closure of our medical school (www.luebeck-kaempft.de).

REFERENCES

1. Colrain IM, Campbell KB. The use of evoked potentials in sleep research. Sleep Med Rev 2007;11(4): 277–93.

2. Rootor DM, Schel JL, Van Dongen HP, et al. Physiological markers of local sleep. Eur J Neurosci 2009; 29(9):1771–8.

3. Priori A. Brain polarization in humans: a reappraisal of an old tool for prolonged non-invasive modulation of brain excitability. Clin Neurophysiol 2003;114(4): 589–95.

4. Iwanovsky A, Dodge C. Electrosleep and electroanesthesia: theory and clinical experience. Foreign Science Bulletin 1968;4:1–64.

5. Brown CC. Electroanesthesia and electrosleep. Am Psychol 1975;30(3):402–10.

6. Nias DK. Therapeutic effects of low-level direct electrical currents. Psychol Bull 1976;83(5):766–73.

7. Kirsch DL, Smith RB. Cranial electrotherapy stimulation for anxiety, depression, insomnia, cognitive dysfunction, and pain: a review and meta-analyses. In: Rosch PJ, Markov MS, editors. Bioelectromagnetic medicine. New York: Marcel Dekker, Inc; 2004. p. 687–99.

8. Dymond AM, Coger RW, Serafetinides EA. Intracerebral current levels in man during electrosleep therapy. Biol Psychiatry 1975;10(1):101–4.

9. Zaghi S, Acar M, Hultgren B, et al. Noninvasive brain stimulation with low-intensity electrical currents: putative mechanisms of action for direct and alternating current stimulation. Neuroscientist 2010; 16(3):285–307.

10. Marshall L, Mölle M, Hallschmid M, et al. Transcranial direct current stimulation during sleep improves declarative memory. J Neurosci 2004;24(44):9985–92.

11. Nitsche MA, Niehaus L, Hoffmann KT, et al. MRI study of human brain exposed to weak direct current stimulation of the frontal cortex. Clin Neurophysiol 2004;115(10):2419–23.

12. Poreisz C, Boros K, Antal A, et al. Safety aspects of transcranial direct current stimulation concerning healthy subjects and patients. Brain Res Bull 2007; 72(4–6):208–14.

13. Vandermeeren Y, Jamart J, Ossemann M. Effect of tDCS with an extracephalic reference electrode on cardio-respiratory and autonomic functions. BMC Neurosci 2010;11:38.

14. Marshall L, Mölle M, Born J. Oscillating current stimulation - slow oscillation stimulation during sleep. Nat Protoc 2006. DOI:10.1038/nprot.2006.299.

15. Huerta PT, Volpe BT. Transcranial magnetic stimulation, synaptic plasticity and network oscillations. J Neuroeng Rehabil 2009;6:7.

16. Wasserman E, Epstein E, Ziemann U. The Oxford handbook of transcranial stimulation. Oxford (UK): Oxford University Press; 2008.

17. Ziemann U, Paulus W, Nitsche MA, et al. Consensus: motor cortex plasticity protocols. Brain Stimul 2008; 1:164–82.

18. Hoogendam JM, Ramakers GM, Di Lazzaro V. Physiology of repetitive transcranial magnetic stimulation of the human brain. Brain Stimul 2010;3(2): 95–118.

19. Wagner T, Fregni F, Fecteau S, et al. Transcranial direct current stimulation: a computer-based human model study. Neuroimage 2007;35(3):1113–24.

20. Wagner T, Eden U, Fregni F, et al. Transcranial magnetic stimulation and brain atrophy: a computer-based human brain model study. Exp Brain Res 2008;186(4):539–50.

21. Datta A, Bansal V, Diaz J, et al. Gyri-precise head model of transcranial direct current stimulation: improved spatial focality using a ring electrode versus conventional rectangular pad. Brain Stimul 2009;2:201–7.

22. Bikson M, Inoue M, Akiyama H, et al. Effects of uniform extracellular DC electric fields on excitability in rat hippocampal slices in vitro. J Physiol 2004; 557(Pt 1):175–90.

23. Nitsche MA, Cohen L, Wasserman E, et al. Transcranial direct current stimulation: state of the art 2008. Brain Stimul 2008;1:206–23.

24. Radman T, Datta A, Ramos RL, et al. One-dimensional representation of a neuron in a uniform electric field. Conf Proc IEEE Eng Med Biol Soc 2009; 2009:6481–4.

25. Thut G, Miniussi C. New insights into rhythmic brain activity from TMS-EEG studies. Trends Cogn Sci 2009;13(4):182–9.

26. Marshall L, Helgadóttir H, Mölle M, et al. Boosting slow oscillations during sleep potentiates memory. Nature 2006;444(7119):610–3.

27. Massimini M, Ferrarelli F, Esser SK, et al. Triggering sleep slow waves by transcranial magnetic stimulation. Proc Natl Acad Sci U S A 2007; 104(20):8496–501.

28. Vyazovskiy VV, Faraguna U, Cirelli C, et al. Triggering slow waves during NREM sleep in the rat by intracortical electrical stimulation: effects of sleep/wake history and background activity. J Neurophysiol 2009;101(4):1921–31.

29. Steriade M, Nunez A, Amzica F. A novel slow (<1 Hz) oscillation of neocortical neurons in vivo: depolarizing and hyperpolarizing components. J Neurosci 1993;13(8):3252–65.

30. Massimini M, Huber R, Ferrarelli F, et al. The sleep slow oscillation as a traveling wave. J Neurosci 2004;24(31):6862–70.

31. Steriade M. Grouping of brain rhythms in corticothalamic systems. Neuroscience 2006;137(4):1087–106.

32. Mölle M, Marshall L, Gais S, et al. Grouping of spindle activity during slow oscillations in human non-rapid eye movement sleep. J Neurosci 2002; 22(24):10941–7.

33. Sirota A, Csicsvari J, Buhl D, et al. Communication between neocortex and hippocampus during sleep in rodents. Proc Natl Acad Sci U S A 2003;100(4):2065–9.

34. Sirota A, Buzsáki G. Interaction between neocortical and hippocampal networks via slow oscillations. Thalamus Relat Syst 2005;3(4):245–59.

35. Lestienne R, Herve-Minvielle A, Robinson D, et al. Slow oscillations as a probe of the dynamics of the locus coeruleus-frontal cortex interaction in anesthetized rats. J Physiol Paris 1997;91(6):273–84.

36. Mölle M, Yeshenko O, Marshall L, et al. Hippocampal sharp wave-ripples linked to slow oscillations in rat slow-wave sleep. J Neurophysiol 2006; 96(1):62–70.

37. Mena-Segovia J, Sims HM, Magill PJ, et al. Cholinergic brainstem neurons modulate cortical gamma activity during slow oscillations. J Physiol 2008; 586(Pt 12):2947–60.

38. Isomura Y, Sirota A, Ozen S, et al. Integration and segregation of activity in entorhinal-hippocampal subregions by neocortical slow oscillations. Neuron 2006;52(5):871–82.

39. Mölle M, Born J. Hippocampus whispering in deep sleep to prefrontal cortex–for good memories? Neuron 2009;61(4):496–8.

40. Massimini M, Rosanova M, Mariotti M. EEG slow (approximately 1 Hz) waves are associated with nonstationarity of thalamo-cortical sensory processing in the sleeping human. J Neurophysiol 2003; 89(3):1205–13.

41. Schroeder CE, Lakatos P. Low-frequency neuronal oscillations as instruments of sensory selection. Trends Neurosci 2009;32(1):9–18.

42. Mazzoni A, Whittingstall K, Brunel N, et al. Understanding the relationships between spike rate and delta/gamma frequency bands of LFPs and EEGs using a local cortical network model. Neuroimage 2009;52(3):956–72.

43. Marshall L, Mölle M, Born J. Spindle and slow wave rhythms at slow wave sleep transitions are linked to strong shifts in the cortical direct current potential. Neuroscience 2003;121(4):1047–53.

44. Marshall L, Born J. The contribution of sleep to hippocampus-dependent memory consolidation. Trends Cogn Sci 2007;11(10):442–50.

45. Fröhlich F, McCormick DA. Endogenous electric fields may guide neocortical network activity. Neuron 2010;67(1):129–43.

46. De Gennaro L, Ferrara M. Sleep spindles: an overview. Sleep Med Rev 2003;7(5):423–40.

47. Himanen SL, Virkkala J, Huhtala H, et al. Spindle frequencies in sleep EEG show U-shape within first four NREM sleep episodes. J Sleep Res 2002; 11(1):35–42.

48. Mölle M, Marshall L, Gais S, et al. Learning increases human electroencephalographic coherence during subsequent slow sleep oscillations. Proc Natl Acad Sci U S A 2004;101(38):13963–8.

49. Kirov R, Weiss C, Siebner HR, et al. Slow oscillation electrical brain stimulation during waking promotes EEG theta activity and memory encoding. Proc Natl Acad Sci U S A 2009;106(36):15460–5.

50. Finelli LA, Baumann H, Borbely AA, et al. Dual electroencephalogram markers of human sleep homeostasis: correlation between theta activity in waking and slow-wave activity in sleep. Neuroscience 2000;101(3):523–9.

51. Vyazovskiy VV, Tobler I. Theta activity in the waking EEG is a marker of sleep propensity in the rat. Brain Res 2005;1050(1–2):64–71.

52. Steenland HW, Wu V, Fukushima H, et al. CaMKIV over-expression boosts cortical 4 7 Hz oscillations during learning and 1–4 Hz delta oscillations during sleep. Mol Brain 2010;3:16.

53. Massimini M, Amzica F. Extracellular calcium fluctuations and intracellular potentials in the cortex during the slow sleep oscillation. J Neurophysiol 2001;85(3):1346–50.

54. Amzica F, Massimini M, Manfridi A. Spatial buffering during slow and paroxysmal sleep oscillations in cortical networks of glial cells in vivo. J Neurosci 2002;22(3):1042–53.

55. Tsukamoto-Yasui M, Sasaki T, Matsumoto W, et al. Active hippocampal networks undergo spontaneous synaptic modification. PLoS One 2007; 2(11):e1250.

56. Wasserman E. Transcranial magnetic stimulation. In: Grafman J, Robertson IH, editors. Handbook of neuropsychology. Plasticity and rehabilitation, vol. 9. 2nd edition. Amsterdam: Elsevier Science B.V; 2003. p. 327–38.

57. Rösler KM. Transcranial magnetic brain stimulation: a tool to investigate central motor pathways. News Physiol Sci 2001;16:297–302.

58. Kujirai T, Caramia MD, Rothwell JC, et al. Corticocortical inhibition in human motor cortex. J Physiol 1993;471:501–19.

59. Ziemann U, Rothwell JC, Ridding MC. Interaction between intracortical inhibition and facilitation in human motor cortex. J Physiol 1996;496(Pt 3):873–81.

60. Hanajima R, Ugawa Y, Terao Y, et al. Paired-pulse magnetic stimulation of the human motor cortex: differences among I waves. J Physiol 1998;509 (Pt 2):607–18.

61. Manganotti P, Fuggetta G, Fiaschi A. Changes of motor cortical excitability in human subjects from wakefulness to early stages of sleep: a combined transcranial magnetic stimulation and electroencephalographic study. Neurosci Lett 2004;362(1):31–4.

62. Grosse P, Khatami R, Salih F, et al. Corticospinal excitability in human sleep as assessed by transcranial magnetic stimulation. Neurology 2002;59(12): 1988–91.

63. Avesani M, Formaggio E, Fuggetta G, et al. Cortico-spinal excitability in human subjects during nonrapid eye movement sleep: single and paired-pulse transcranial magnetic stimulation study. Exp Brain Res 2008;187(1):17–23.

64. Salih F, Khatami R, Steinheimer S, et al. Inhibitory and excitatory intracortical circuits across the human sleep-wake cycle using paired-pulse transcranial magnetic stimulation. J Physiol 2005;565 (Pt 2):695–701.

65. Salih F, Khatami R, Steinheimer S, et al. A hypothesis for how non-REM sleep might promote seizures in partial epilepsies: a transcranial magnetic stimulation study. Epilepsia 2007;48(8):1538–42.

66. De Gennaro L, Bertini M, Ferrara M, et al. Intracortical inhibition and facilitation upon awakening from different sleep stages: a transcranial magnetic stimulation study. Eur J Neurosci 2004;19(11):3099–104.

67. Balkin TJ, Braun AR, Wesensten NJ, et al. The process of awakening: a PET study of regional brain activity patterns mediating the re-establishment of alertness and consciousness. Brain 2002;125(Pt 10): 2308–19.

68. Bergmann TO, Mölle M, Schmidt MA, et al. EEG-triggered transcranial magnetic stimulation reveals motor cortical excitability changes during up- and down-states of the human sleep slow oscillation. ESRS, September, 2010.

69. Bergmann TO, Groppa S, Seeger M, et al. Acute changes in motor cortical excitability during slow oscillatory and constant anodal transcranial direct current stimulation. J Neurophysiol 2009;102(4):2303–11.

70. Gao L, Meng X, Ye C, et al. Entrainment of slow oscillations of auditory thalamic neurons by repetitive sound stimuli. J Neurosci 2009;29(18):6013–21.

71. Van Der Werf YD, Altena E, Schoonheim MM, et al. Sleep benefits subsequent hippocampal functioning. Nat Neurosci 2009;12(2):122–3.

72. Plihal W, Born J. Effects of early and late nocturnal sleep on declarative and procedural memory. J Cogn Neurosci 1997;9(4):534–47.

73. Wagner U, Gais S, Born J. Emotional memory formation is enhanced across sleep intervals with high amounts of rapid eye movement sleep. Learn Mem 2001;8(2):112–9.

74. Gais S, Born J. Declarative memory consolidation: mechanisms acting during human sleep. Learn Mem 2004;11(6):679–85.

75. Clemens Z, Mölle M, Eross L, et al. Temporal coupling of parahippocampal ripples, sleep spindles and slow oscillations in humans. Brain 2007; 130(Pt 11):2868–78.

76. Mölle M, Eschenko O, Gais S, et al. The influence of learning on sleep slow oscillations and associated spindles and ripples in humans and rats. Eur J Neurosci 2009;29(5):1071–81.

77. Buzsáki G. Two-stage model of memory trace formation: a role for "noisy" brain states. Neuroscience 1989;31(3):551–70.

78. Buzsáki G. The hippocampo-neocortical dialogue. Cereb Cortex 1996;6(2):81–92.

79. Wierzynski CM, Lubenov EV, Gu M, et al. State-dependent spike-timing relationships between hippocampal and prefrontal circuits during sleep. Neuron 2009;61(4):587–96.

80. Girardeau G, Benchenane K, Wiener SI, et al. Selective suppression of hippocampal ripples impairs spatial memory. Nat Neurosci 2009;12(10):1222–3.

81. Rechtschaffen A, Kales A. A manual of standardized terminology, techniques and scoring system for sleep stages of human subjects. Washington, DC: NIH Publ. 204, US Government Printing Office; 1968.

82. Allen EA, Pasley BN, Duong T, et al. Transcranial magnetic stimulation elicits coupled neural and hemodynamic consequences. Science 2007; 317(5846):1918–21.

83. Merzagora AC, Foffani G, Panyavin I, et al. Prefrontal hemodynamic changes produced by anodal direct current stimulation. Neuroimage 2010;49(3):2304–10.

84. Stagg CJ, Best JG, Stephenson MC, et al. Polarity-sensitive modulation of cortical neurotransmitters by transcranial stimulation. J Neurosci 2009;29(16): 5202–6.

85. Yoon EJ, Kim YK, Lee HS, et al. Evaluation of tDCS effect on regional cerebral glucose metabolism in patients with central pain. J Nucl Med 2009; 50(Suppl 2):1276.

86. Uhlhaas PJ, Singer W. Neural synchrony in brain disorders: relevance for cognitive dysfunctions and pathophysiology. Neuron 2006;52(1):155–68.

87. Giuditta A, Ambrosini MV, Montagnese P, et al. The sequential hypothesis of the function of sleep. Behav Brain Res 1995;69(1–2):157–66.

88. Ribeiro S, Nicolelis MA. Reverberation, storage, and postsynaptic propagation of memories during sleep. Learn Mem 2004;11(6):686–96.

89. Diekelmann S, Born J. The memory function of sleep. Nat Rev Neurosci 2010;11(2):114–26.

90. Bergmann TO, Molle M, Marshall L, et al. A local signature of LTP- and LTD-like plasticity in human NREM sleep. Eur J Neurosci 2008;27(9):2241–9.

91. De GL, Fratello F, Marzano C, et al. Cortical plasticity induced by transcranial magnetic stimulation during wakefulness affects electroencephalogram activity during sleep. PLoS One 2008;3(6):e2483.

92. Huber R, Maatta S, Esser SK, et al. Measures of cortical plasticity after transcranial paired associative stimulation predict changes in electroencephalogram slow-wave activity during subsequent sleep. J Neurosci 2008;28(31):7911–8.

93. Weiss SA, Faber DS. Field effects in the CNS play functional roles. Front Neural Circuits 2010;4:15.

Memory, Sleep, and Dreaming: Experiencing Consolidation

Erin J. Wamsley, PhD[a], Robert Stickgold, PhD[b],*

KEYWORDS
- Sleep • Memory • Dreaming • Mentation • Cognition
- Consolidation • Default network • Resting states

During all stages of sleep, the mind and brain are working to process new memories, consolidating them into long-term storage and integrating recently acquired information with past experience. In recent years, an accumulating body of research evidence has definitively shown that postlearning sleep is beneficial for human memory performance across a variety of tasks, including verbal learning,[1-4] procedural skill learning,[2,5-7] emotional memory,[8,9] and spatial navigation.[10,11] Memories of recent experience appear nightly in the content of our dreams, and animal research shows that presleep experience is replayed on a cellular level during postlearning sleep. Sleep-dependent memory consolidation has been extensively examined from a variety of behavioral and neuroscientific perspectives, but studies examining dream experience as an indicator of mnemonic activity in the sleeping brain are conspicuously absent. This article reviews evidence that the use of subjective report as a method for probing the activities of the mind and brain is critical for a comprehensive approach to understanding memory consolidation. Recent work suggests that dream experiences recalled from sleep are a direct reflection of concomitant memory processes in the brain.

MEMORIES IN THE SLEEPING BRAIN
The Reactivation and Consolidation of Memory during Sleep

There is strong evidence that at least one function of sleep is to consolidate fragile new memory traces into more permanent forms of long-term storage, integrating key features of recent experience with existing remote and semantic memory networks. Behavioral studies in humans have clearly shown that postlearning sleep is beneficial for memory performance in a variety of learning domains. Until recently, much of this work focused on simple procedural tasks, showing that basic motor and perceptual skills were optimally developed across posttraining periods that included sleep, relative to equivalent periods of wakefulness. Accumulating data now also strongly implicate sleep in the consolidation of various forms of complex declarative memory, similarly showing that relative to wakefulness, sleep after learning leads to superior memory performance at later test.

Models of the brain processes supporting these mnemonic benefits of sleep have drawn heavily from animal literature showing a neural-level reactivation of recent experience during periods of posttraining sleep and quiet rest. Initially focusing on the hippocampus, this literature has now

a Department of Psychiatry, Harvard Medical School/Beth Israel Deaconess Medical Center, 330 Brookline Avenue, E/FD 862, Boston, MA 02215, USA
b Department of Psychiatry, Harvard Medical School/Beth Israel Deaconess Medical Center, 330 Brookline Avenue, E/FD 861, Boston, MA 02215, USA
* Corresponding author.
E-mail address: rstickgold@hms.harvard.edu

Sleep Med Clin 6 (2011) 97–108
doi:10.1016/j.jsmc.2010.12.008
1556-407X/11/$ – see front matter © 2011 Elsevier Inc. All rights reserved.

shown that across a wide network of brain systems, patterns of neural activity that are first seen when waking animals are exploring an environment are later reproduced when these animals sleep. This reactivation has most consistently been observed during periods of nonrapid eye movement (NREM) sleep just after learning, during brief hippocampal sharp-wave ripple burst events[12,13] (**Fig. 1**A). This replay of memory in sleep may be critical to long-term memory consolidation. In direct support of this hypothesis, a recent study has shown that the extent of neural pattern reactivation after learning predicts subsequent gains in memory performance.[14] Human neurophysiologic studies have linked consolidation to sleep-specific electrophysiologic and neurochemical events, and have used functional imaging technologies to show a systems-level reactivation of brain regions active in encoding new memories (**Fig. 1**B), roughly analogous to that which has been seen in rodents.

Classically, the consolidation of memory has been conceptualized as a process of strengthening an initially labile memory trace, such that the new memory is rendered increasingly resistant to interference across time. Much of the literature on sleep and memory has thus focused on simple quantitative measures of memory strength (eg, the

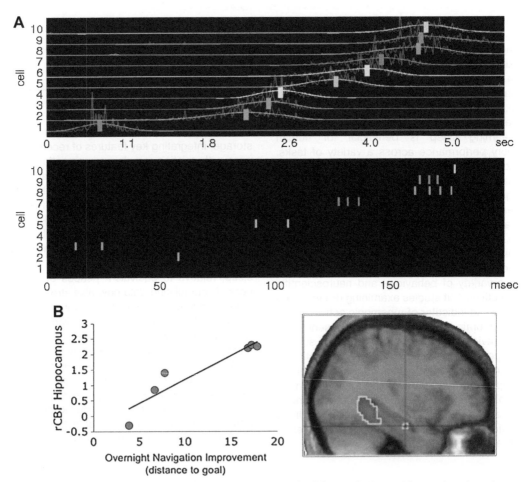

Fig. 1. (*A*) In animals, memory reactivation is seen as patterns of cell firings during waking exploration of an environment (*top*) that are reiterated in subsequent NREM sleep (*bottom*), albeit on a faster timescale. Vertical bars represent the time of peak firing for 10 individual cells, showing clear place fields in the training environment. (*B*) In humans, evidence of reactivation has been reported in imaging studies, showing that brain regions engaged during task encoding are again active during posttraining sleep. In this example, reactivation of hippocampal activity during posttraining sleep (*right*) predicted overnight improvement in memory performance on a spatial learning task (*left*). (*Adapted from* Lee AK, Wilson MA. Memory of sequential experience in the hippocampus during slow wave sleep. Neuron 2002;1186; with permission; and Peigneux P, Laureys S, Fuchs S, et al. Are spatial memories strengthened in the human hippocampus during slow wave sleep? Neuron 2004;541; with permission.)

number of words recalled, or the number of motor sequences completed). However, it is becoming clear that the role of sleep is more complex than strengthening memories in their original forms. To the contrary, recent studies have shown that sleep is important for such complex processes as the integration of new information into established cortical memory networks,[15,16] the extraction of meaning,[17] and the development of insight.[18] Recent studies by Dumay and Gaskell[16] and Tamminen and colleagues[15] describe the first of these concepts. As newly learned words become integrated into neocortical lexical networks over time, competition with previously known words develops, and this competition can be measured as slowed reaction times to those well-known words that are similar to the newly acquired words. In a lexical integration paradigm, participants learn a set of pseudowords that are phonemically similar to well-known words (eg, cathedruke is a pseudoword similar to the word cathedral) and response times to the new and old words are measured. Dumay and Gaskell[16] have reported that competition between new and existing words emerges only after a period of sleep, thus suggesting that newly learned words are integrated into neocortical lexical networks by sleep-dependent processes. Using the same task, Tamminen and colleagues[15] found that the degree of lexical integration over a night of sleep is associated with sleep spindles.

A recent study from our own laboratory suggests that sleep functions to transform memories such that the critical gist of an experience is retained, whereas specific details of the material are discarded. In the Deese-Roediger-McDermott paradigm, participants learn several lists of semantically related words. At a delayed test, when participants are asked to recall these words, often they also report having seen "gist" words, which describe the general theme of the memorized word lists, but which were not themselves present in the list. Sleep preferentially benefited (false) memory for these gist words, suggesting that one function of sleep-dependent memory processing is to extract meaningful generalities from large collections of related memories.[17] These and other recent studies suggest that sleep functions not simply to strengthen memories, but in addition to transform memory traces by integrating them into mnemonic networks and preferentially maintaining the general meaning or gist of the larger experience.

In parallel with this behavioral work, human brain imaging studies have described a sleep-dependent reorganization of the network of brain structures supporting subsequent recall.[19–22] For example, for hippocampus-dependent declarative memories, retrieval-associated activity in the hippocampal complex decreases after sleep, whereas related activation in cortical structures, particularly medial prefrontal areas, increases.[19,20] Such evidence supports models of systems-level declarative memory consolidation proposing that memory retrieval, although initially dependent on the hippocampus for retrieval, becomes increasingly less reliant on the hippocampal system and more reliant on cortical structures over time,[23] and that this developing hippocampal independence may occur during sleep. Other functional magnetic resonance imaging (fMRI) studies have described an analogous sleep-dependent reorganization of emotional memory, such that medial prefrontal structures become more engaged at delayed retrieval when participants have been allowed to sleep immediately after encoding, in concert with increased retrieval-related functional connectivity between cortical and subcortical regions involved in emotional memory processing.[21,22] This type of functional memory reorganization, in which hippocampally dependent memories are gradually reencoded into cortical networks that rely on strongly overlapping and related representations, could underlie the ability of sleep to facilitate both the integration of recent memory with past experience and the abstraction of general concepts from specific stimulus material.

Linking Sleep-dependent Memory Processing with Dream Experience

Given that humans dream, the neurophysiologic and fMRI evidence that memories are reactivated during sleep suggests that replay of experience in the sleeping brain could be related to the conscious experience of dreaming. Several key features of sleep-dependent memory reactivation and consolidation strongly parallel the form in which recently encoded memory appears in sleep mentation. These parallels are introduced in this section and expanded on in later sections.

First, qualitatively different types of memory seem to be processed preferentially during different stages of human sleep. Hippocampus-dependent memory, for example, seems to benefit particularly from NREM sleep, perhaps especially slow wave sleep (SWS), whereas memory for emotional material may be preferentially enhanced by rapid eye movement (REM) sleep. Mirroring these proposed mnemonic functions of REM and NREM sleep, characteristics of dream experience vary similarly as a function of sleep stage. For example, subjective reports elicited from NREM sleep stages are more likely to contain episodic memory sources (a hippocampus-dependent form of memory) than are reports from REM sleep,[24] whereas dream experiences from REM sleep are unique in the presence of particularly intense emotions.[25]

Second, a prominent feature of memory reactivation in rodent models is that, within NREM sleep, the strength of neural-level memory replay decays quickly across time.[26,27] Similarly, it seems that sleep mentation may be most strongly related to recent memories early in the sleep phase,[24,28,29] with this association to recent experience decreasing over time.

Earlier, we also introduced the concept that sleep transforms human memories, rather than veridically strengthening them. Both rodent neural reactivation studies and data on human dreaming support this notion that recent experience is not faithfully replayed in videotapelike fashion during sleep. Neuronal firing sequences established during wake are reexpressed only intermittently during rodent NREM sleep, with low fidelity and on a faster timescale than the original experience.[30,31] Similarly, only intermittent fragments of recent episodic memories appear in sleep mentation, intermingled with remote and semantically related material.[29,32]

Third, there are several key features of the organization of the sleeping brain believed to play a critical role in supporting both offline memory processing and the formation of dream experience. As we fall asleep, the brain quickly undergoes dramatic changes in functional activation patterns, and in the composition of the neurochemical/neurohormone milieu driving the system. During all stages of sleep, regional cerebral blood flow to a network of frontal areas is dramatically decreased, relative to waking,[33] whereas activity in a network of memory-related areas, including the hippocampal complex, medial prefrontal cortex, and anterior cingulate, remains relatively increased during both REM and NREM sleep stages. As we enter early-night NREM-dominated sleep, levels of acetylcholine are dramatically reduced relative to waking, so that monoaminergic neurotransmitters dominate the system. These low levels of acetylcholine during NREM sleep have been hypothesized to facilitate the offline consolidation of hippocampus-dependent memory,[34] during a time at which recent episodic memories are most likely to be appearing in concomitant dream experience.[24,29] Reduced levels of cortisol during early night, SWS-dominated sleep have also been hypothesized to both facilitate hippocampal-cortical interactions underlying memory consolidation[35,36] and to promote brain dynamics supporting NREM-type dream experience.[36]

Recent papers in sleep and memory have liberally speculated on a possible connection between sleep-dependent memory processing on the one hand, and the imagery, thoughts, and feelings comprising dream experience on the other.[30,36–40] Most recently, observations that the replay of memory in sleeping rodents occurs not only in the hippocampus but in sensory cortices as well have seemed to offer empirical evidence that "the expression of these reactivated memory traces in sensory cortex may directly relate to the perceptual imagery experienced during sleep and dream states."[30] However, the presence of memory-related brain activity during sleep does not necessarily imply that this activity is consciously experienced, and hence does not imply a relationship to dream experiences recalled from this period of sleep. Until recently, little empirical work has attempted to directly test the hypothesis that dream experience reflects the reactivation and consolidation of specific mnemonic content in the sleeping brain. Before describing these studies, we consider the nature of incorporation of recent experiences into sleep mentation more generally, and describe how these observations can inform our approach to understanding offline memory consolidation processes.

THE INCORPORATION OF RECENT EXPERIENCE INTO DREAMING

Recent memories constitute a significant component of sleep mentation. In 1900, Freud[41] coined the term "day residue" to describe the presence of recent life experience in dream content, a phenomenon which he viewed as only secondary in relevance to the true latent meaning of a dream. But as the notion that dreams harbor a secret meaning decipherable only by trained psychoanalysts has fallen into disfavor, it has become increasingly clear that the appearance of newly encoded information in our daydreams, mental imagery, thoughts, and dreams may be an observation of paramount importance to understanding the activities of mind and brain during both wake and sleep. The form in which memories are incorporated into dream experience in many ways parallels what we know about memory consolidation during sleep, and may help us to understand the process of long-term memory consolidation.

Effects of Presleep Experience on Sleep Mentation

In the 1960s and 1970s, a considerable amount of research effort was devoted to understanding the relation of waking events to dream content by manipulating participants' presleep experience.

Despite methodological weaknesses that plagued much of this literature, several useful conclusions can be drawn from this early work. Most notable is the extreme difficulty of manipulating dream content, even when highly emotional stimuli are introduced before sleep. Of the dozens of such studies performed during this time,[42–47] almost none showed unambiguous, statistically significant effects of an experimentally introduced presleep stimulus on subsequent dream content. The most consistently observed effect of waking experience on laboratory-collected sleep mentation has been a powerful influence of the laboratory setting itself. For example, in an analysis of 813 REM mentation reports collected across several studies, Dement and colleagues[48] reported that 22% of reports unambiguously incorporated either isolated elements of the laboratory situation (eg, the experimenter, electrodes) or more complete representations of the experimental setting (ie, a combination of these elements). In retrospect, given the salience of sleeping in a strange place and being awakened during the night to report dreams, it is hardly surprising that the laboratory environment overshadows the effect of any particular film or activity introduced as part of an experimental protocol. In contrast, more recent data from our own laboratory, discussed later, show that experimental introduction of intensive and engaging learning experiences can dramatically influence the content of dreaming, at least early in the night.

Other, nonexperimental approaches provide solid empirical evidence that the content of sleep mentation often references new memories and recent experiences. For example, in an analysis comparing 299 home-collected dream reports with possible memory sources from a diary of waking events, Fosse and colleagues[32] reported that fragments of recent experience are often seen in dreams. Although exact replication of any particular waking experience was rare, 51% of reports were judged to contain at least one dream element bearing strong similarity to a recent waking experience. Other research has similarly prompted participants to connect dream reports with likely memory sources from waking experience in the previous days and weeks,[24,49–51] showing that such memory sources are readily identified with high confidence, and correspond with the ratings of blind judges.[49] We return later to this notion that recent experience appears in sleep mentation in a fragmentary form, rather than as an exact videotapelike replay of an event.

Other lines of work have explored the more general correspondence between sleep mentation and waking life. In collaboration with Robert Van de Castle, Calvin Hall[52] pioneered the use of content analysis methods to quantitatively assess the content of large sets of mentation reports. A response to the methodological pitfalls inherent in subjective interpretations of dream content used by psychoanalysts, this meticulous classification system counts the occurrence of different types of characters, settings, objects, social interactions, activities, and so forth, explicitly described in the text of mentation reports. Using this system, Hall illustrated the transparent relationship between dream content and everyday life by creating surprisingly accurate profiles and histories of psychiatric patients based solely on blind content analysis of dream reports, and became amongst the first to champion the notion that quantitative methods could uncover straightforward and meaningful relationships between waking experience and dream content.

"A large number of dreams reflect faithfully the daytime activities and preoccupations of the dreamer. Skiers dream of skiing, surfers dream of surfing, and mountain climbers dream of climbing mountains. Teachers dream of classroom situations, bankers dream of banking activities, and nurses dream about their patients."[53]

More recent applications of Hall's system of content analysis have reported consistent, statistically significant differences in dream content of groups of individuals with divergent waking experience (ie, between males and females, children and adults, blind and sighted individuals [for a review, see Ref.[54]]). These investigations have contributed to our understanding of the dreaming process by reminding us that, although attempts to predict or control dream content have often failed, a broad correspondence between sleep mentation and waking experience is nonetheless transparently obvious.

Determinants of the Memory Sources of Dreaming

But what determines which memories contribute to the content of dreaming on a particular night? Far from being a haphazard process, the incorporation of waking experience into sleep mentation seems to follow a set of predictable patterns, modulated by both sleep stage and temporal distance from a waking event. Contrary to the entrenched popular belief that REM sleep = dreaming, we dream during all stages of sleep.[55–58] Although reports of mental experiences from NREM sleep stages 2, 3, and 4 are often shorter and less emotional than REM reports, there is considerable overlap in the cognitive characteristics of reports from different stages of sleep (eg, see Ref.[59]). Late-night NREM dreaming can be just as vivid, bizarre, and storylike as the typical dream from REM sleep.[57,60] Yet one consistent difference between dream reports from different stages of sleep seems to be the nature of participant-identified memory sources. Coinciding with the notion that NREM dreams tend to be more realistic and mundane than reports from REM sleep, mentation reports from NREM stages are characterized by a large proportion of episodic memory sources,[24] derived from memories of specific autobiographical events that occurred at a particular place and time. Dream reports from REM sleep, on the other hand, incorporate more abstract and semantic memory sources, unrelated to specific life events. Thus, during NREM sleep a participant might report a dream concerning a friend she saw the previous afternoon, whereas dreams during later REM sleep would likely be more bizarre and not obviously connected to any specific presleep experience.

The incorporation of recent experience into dream content also seems to follow an organized temporal pattern. Very recent events are more often incorporated into mentation occurring early in the sleep phase, with remote experiences appearing only later in the night. Although only a few studies have examined time-of-night effects on incorporation in this manner, both the recency of subject-identified memory sources[61] and the similarity of sleep mentation reports to presleep thought[62] have been reported to correlate negatively with time since sleep onset. Work from our own laboratory using engaging video game learning tasks has shown that incidence of direct, unambiguous incorporation of task-related imagery at sleep onset declines linearly as a function of time since the initiation of sleep.[28,29] On a broader timescale, it seems that recent life events are most likely to appear in dream content, relative to more remote experiences from years past.[63,64] Several studies also suggest that waking experiences tend to be incorporated into dream mentation either immediately after the experience, or else about a week later (the dream lag effect[49,65]).

These observations lead us to conclude that NREM sleep early in the night is the state of sleep most likely to contain replay of recent memory. As described earlier, this notion is supported by the animal literature, in which neuronal-level memory reactivation has typically been observed during periods of NREM sleep immediately after learning, with the strength of this replay decaying rapidly across time. In contrast, only a single study has reported similar reactivation of memory during REM sleep.[39] Our recent work examining the effects of learning tasks on sleep mentation have thus focused on periods of stage 1 and 2 NREM sleep immediately after sleep onset.

The Effects of Intensive Learning Experiences on Sleep Onset Mentation

Studies in our own laboratory have examined NREM sleep mentation after intensive training on engaging, video-gamelike tasks. Concentrating on periods of early night NREM sleep, this research shows that salient, interactive learning tasks can exert a dramatic influence on subsequent sleep mentation. In one such study, participants played the video game Tetris extensively several hours before sleep.[28] When mentation reports were then repeatedly elicited after short intervals of sleep, 64% of participants reported unambiguous game-related images in at least one sleep onset report. In a related investigation using a downhill skiing arcade game,[29] 30% of all posttraining mentation reports directly incorporated the game (**Fig. 2**). The frequency of direct incorporation in these sleep onset studies, dramatically higher than that observed in any previous overnight investigation, suggests that the first minutes of sleep provide ideal conditions for the cognitive-level reactivation of waking experience. Furthermore, it may be that interactive learning experiences are more likely to be reactivated as participants fall asleep than are passively viewed experimental stimuli.

Interleaved Fragments of Experience

Despite the strong influence of waking experience on subsequent sleep mentation, dreams rarely consist of an exact replay of a life event. Instead, sleep mentation incorporates isolated elements of a waking episode, intermingled with fragments of other recent memories, as well as remote and semantic memory material, thus creating novel and sometimes bizarre scenarios that do not faithfully represent any particular waking event. For example, the following illustrates a sleep onset dream report that clearly incorporates fragments of a waking experience, but without replicating the original context in which these fragments were embedded (data from Ref.[32]).

Waking experience
When I left [work at] Starbucks, we had so many leftover pastries and muffins to throw away or take home, I couldn't decide which muffins to take and which to toss …

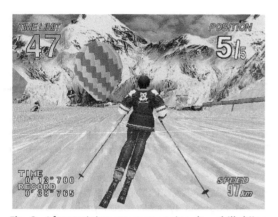

Fig. 2. After training on an engaging downhill skiing arcade game, 30% of 386 sleep onset mentation reports contained task-related imagery or thoughts. Representation of the game primarily took the form of sensory imagery as opposed to thought, and most often bore a direct, unambiguous relationship to the game. Examples of direct incorporation: "I get like flashes of that … game in my head, virtual reality skiing game … downhill umm race, in my head. Umm, there's this one particular corner that I haven't quite been able to master, and every time I get flashes of it, it's like that corner that umm I keep crashing into in my head." "I once again, saw the, the game, it was smooth at first, and then it went into the cave, and then it just stopped like abruptly, like the game turned off." Examples of indirect incorporation: "I was picturing stacking wood this time … I felt like I was doing it at … at a ski resort that I had been to before, like 5 years ago maybe." "I was in a race. Um, like a running race, um … sort of like through San Francisco. It was kind of hilly and it wasn't difficult. Like, I was just kind of coasting through the race I think." (*Adapted from* Wamsley EJ, Perry K, Djonlagic I, et al. Cognitive replay of visuo-motor learning at sleep onset: temporal dynamics and relationship to task performance. Sleep 2010;33:59; with permission.)

Corresponding sleep mentation

My dad and I leave to go shopping. We go from room to room, store to store. One of the stores is filled with muffins, muffins, muffins from floor to ceiling, all different kinds, I can't decide which one I want …

In studies of sleep onset and stage 2 NREM sleep reports after playing video games,[28,29] we have similarly observed that, rather than faithfully reiterating a learning task, mentation reports integrated elements of the learning experience into a narrative that included related material drawn from remote and semantic memory. For example, after training on a downhill skiing arcade game,[29] one participant reported at sleep onset, "I was picturing stacking wood this time … I felt like I

was doing it at … at a ski resort that I had been to before, like 5 years ago maybe.." Similarly, after training on a virtual maze navigation task,[66] a participant reported "I was thinking about the maze and kinda having people as check points, I guess, and then that led me to think about when I went on this trip a few years ago and we went to see these bat caves, and they're kind of like, mazelike." Thus, when incorporated into a dream, the various components of a wake episode do not seem to remain bound together in the way that characterizes the mental time travel of episodic memory recall in waking life.

This observation that dreams do not veridically replay waking experience has led some to conclude that such mental activity is incompatible with consolidation of memory.[67,68] To the contrary, emerging evidence suggests that the fragmentary form in which waking experience appears in dreams, intermingled with other memory traces, reflects a critical feature of the memory consolidation process. As described earlier, consolidation seems to be considerably more complex than the strengthening of memories in their original forms, and the neuronal-level memory reactivation described in animals does not consist of a precise, veridical reiteration of waking experience. Instead, patterns of neural activity that statistically resemble (but are not identical to) those established in waking experience are played out on a speeded timescale. Furthermore, when animals are exposed to 2 successive spatial experiences, reactivation of both patterns seems to be instantiated simultaneously during subsequent NREM sleep.[26] Compatible with this observation is the proposal that sleep functions to transform memory traces in part by slowly interleaving neural representations of recent experience into existing remote and semantic cortical networks.[38,69] For example, in their influential article in *Psychological Review*, McClelland and colleagues speculate that optimal consolidation of new memories requires the alternating reactivation of these memories and related remote memories during different stages of sleep:

Once a memory is stored in the hippocampal system, it can be reactivated and then reinstated in the neocortex … [R]einstatement provides the opportunity for an incremental adjustment of neocortical connections, thereby allowing memories initially dependent on the hippocampal system to gradually become independent of it. We assume that reinstatement also occurs in off-line situations, including active rehearsal, reminiscence, and other inactive states including sleep ... Possibly, events reactivated in the hippocampus during slow wave sleep prime related neocortical patterns, so that these in turn become available for activation during REM sleep. This could permit both new and old information to be played back in closely interleaved fashion.[69]

Following this line of reasoning, we propose that even within a single dream experience, sleep mentation reflects the interleaved reactivation of memory fragments from different recent and remote sources, allowing newly acquired information to become increasingly connected with related memory traces across time. By initiating long-term potentiation–like plasticity in mnemonic networks, this simple process of simultaneously activating new and old memory traces during sleep could account for behavioral data indicating that sleep facilitates the integration of new information with existing semantic networks,[15,16] as well as the extraction of meaning,[17] which may require a similar process of relating new information to existing knowledge. However, despite many hypotheses relating the conscious experience of dreaming to memory processing, this notion is yet to be subjected to systematic empirical investigation.

THE EMPIRICAL STUDY OF SPONTANEOUS SUBJECTIVE EXPERIENCE

For the most part, cognitive neuroscience has abandoned the behaviorist notion that conscious, subjective experience is not a suitable object for empirical investigation. Research in the last 2 decades has moved beyond the philosophic question of mind-brain relationship and begun in earnest to study the neural correlates, for example, of motivation, emotion, attention, mental imagery, and episodic memory. Often, mapping the brain basis of these subjective concepts relies on taking participants' verbal reports of experience at face value. Yet neuroscience has been slow to formalize the study of spontaneous subjective experience during offline states, when responses to sensory stimuli no longer drive the system. Although research on the default mode of brain function has brought attention to the importance of spontaneous brain activity occurring during periods of rest and sleep,[70,71] virtually none of this work has examined participants' own reports of what is going through their mind at rest. Data on spontaneous cognition during sleep have been even more lacking. Neurophysiologic studies seeking to shed light on the neural basis of dreaming have often relied merely on describing the physiology of REM, or else have dichotomized conscious experience as either present or absent, without exploring the content of this mentation.

Earlier, we argued that the specific content of conscious experience during sleep (whether termed sleep mentation, dreaming, or hypnagogic imagery) is clearly relevant to understanding memory consolidation. Yet despite widespread theoretic agreement that sleep-dependent memory processing may relate to dream experience,[30,36–40,72] attempts to empirically address this hypothesis have been conspicuously absent. Why? First, for historical reasons, dream experience has typically been presumed to be difficult or impossible to quantify in a scientifically rigorous manner. Psychoanalytic approaches entrenched in the popular imagination have characterized dreaming as a mysterious, symbolic form of mental activity that, unlike waking cognition, cannot be measured, classified, and quantitatively analyzed in a meaningful way. Pseudoscientific approaches to dreaming popularized in the media have created a perception that, when occurring during sleep, cognition is not a legitimate area of scientific inquiry. This is not the case. There is little, if any, evidence that conscious experience during sleep is particularly more inaccessible, complex, or symbolic than waking thought. Furthermore, reliable approaches to quantifying dream content have been available for decades,[52,59] and methods of data collection are straightforward and completely compatible with standard designs in memory research. Although memory for sleep mentation is typically more fleeting than for waking experience, all self-report measures, whether for waking or sleep mentation, rely on taking post hoc reports of unverifiable data at face value ("Did you see the stimulus?" "What strategy did you use to encode the material?" "To what degree have the following symptoms bothered you in the past month?"). Resurgent studies of such subjective concepts as emotion, mood, memory, and belief show the progress that can be made when one takes a simple and straightforward approach to subjective experience, casting obfuscating philosophic concerns aside.

Critically, the content of spontaneous subjective experience can provide information inaccessible via any other means. The use of subjective report is an ideal method to determine whether a specific memory is being reactivated in the sleeping brain. Particularly in human research, there is no known measure of brain activity (eg, electroencephalography, fMRI, positron emission tomography) that can convincingly show the activation of a specific memory. For example, increased regional cerebral blood flow to learning-related brain regions suggests that the same memory systems engaged at learning are doing something during sleep, but does not show the reactivation of a particular memory. Conscious retrieval of a recent memory, in contrast, definitely shows that the neural networks encoding that particular memory have been reactivated. Subjective reports allow us a detailed view of the form in which a memory is retrieved. For example, as described earlier, reports of sleep mentation reveal that recent memory fragments are reactivated in an interleaved fashion with past experience and semantic knowledge. Such observations illuminate how the brain transforms memories over time by integrating recently acquired information into existing knowledge structures. Reports of conscious experience are unique in enabling us to explore which memories of everyday waking experience are spontaneously reactivated during offline states of quiet rest and sleep.

REACTIVATION OF MEMORY IN DREAM CONTENT AND SLEEP-DEPENDENT MEMORY CONSOLIDATION

Although empirical investigation of these questions has been largely lacking, a handful of studies provide noteworthy evidence for a link between learning, sleep-dependent memory consolidation, and dream experience. That dreaming might function to process previous experience is a hypothesis predating the current resurgence of interest in sleep-dependent memory consolidation, and several studies from the 1960s onwards have addressed this question. Fiss and colleagues[73] investigated the morning recall of short stories encoded the night before, finding a correlation between story-related words in dream reports and memory for these stories the following morning. De Koninck and colleagues[74,75] have also examined the correlation between sleep mentation and verbal learning, exploring dream content as a corollary of language learning in an academic setting. Amongst students enrolled in a French-immersion language class, those who showed superior acquisition of the new language across a 6-week course tended to incorporate French into dream content more often than students who were less successful in the class.[74,75] Hypothesizing that REM sleep dreaming is important for emotional adaptation to stressful events, the work of Rosalind Cartwright has examined dream content as a predictor of psychological outcomes in women after divorce, finding that characteristics of spouse-related dreams predict remission from depression.[76] Other work also supports a role for sleep in emotional adaptation to negative experiences.[77,78]

Recent work from our own laboratory has provided direct evidence that incorporation of a learning task into subsequent dream experience predicts enhanced sleep-dependent memory consolidation.[66] In this study, participants were trained on a three-dimensional style virtual maze task (**Fig. 3**, left) before an opportunity for a 1.5-hour nap or else for an equivalent period of wake. During this period, all subjects were

A

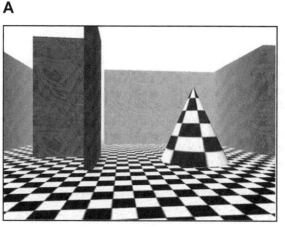

B

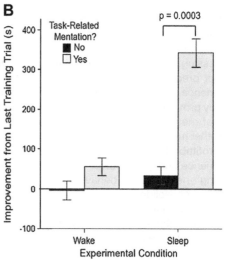

Fig. 3. (A, B) Dreaming of a spatial learning task is associated with enhanced navigation performance at delayed retest, whereas thinking of the task during wakefulness is unrelated to later performance. Error bars represent ± standard error of the mean. (*Adapted from* Wamsley EJ, Tucker M, Payne JD, et al. Dreaming of a learning task is associated with enhanced sleep-dependent memory consolidation. Curr Biol 2010;20:850; with permission.)

prompted 3 times to make open-ended verbal reports of "everything that was going through your mind." We found that reports of task-related mentation were strongly associated with enhanced performance at subsequent retest (**Fig. 3**, right). In the sleep group, participants who spontaneously referred to the maze task in their subjective reports improved 10-fold more at retest than sleep participants who gave no task-related reports ($P = .0003$). In contrast, thinking of the maze while awake did not provide any performance benefit (condition × mentation interaction: $P = .08$). These findings show how reports of subjective experience can inform the study of memory consolidation, providing novel evidence that dream experience reflects the learning-induced reactivation of memory networks during sleep, and that such reactivation correlates with substantially enhanced memory performance.

SUMMARY

Recent advances in our understanding of long-term memory processing suggest that after learning, waking experience is reactivated in the sleeping brain, leading to a process of consolidation by which new, labile memory traces are reorganized into more permanent forms of long-term storage. Dream experiences recalled from sleep bear a transparent relationship to recently encoded information, and provide a useful window into consolidation-related activities of the sleeping brain. Recent work from our laboratory has established a direct relationship between the replay of recent experience in dream content, and enhanced memory performance in humans.[66]

We have argued here that the study of spontaneous conscious experience has great potential for elucidating the mechanisms of offline memory processing, particularly by allowing an examination of precisely which memories from everyday experience are reactivated during offline states, and by providing detailed information on the activities of memory systems that is not available by any other means. It is our hope that future research will profitably focus on the quantification of subject experience during periods of quiet rest and sleep, relating neural and behavioral measures of memory consolidation to the particular form in which new information is incorporated into dreaming, interleaved with established remote and semantic memory networks.

REFERENCES

1. Ellenbogen JM, Hulbert JC, Stickgold R, et al. Interfering with theories of sleep and memory: sleep, declarative memory, and associative interference. Curr Biol 2006;16:1290.

2. Plihal W, Born J. Effects of early and late nocturnal sleep on declarative and procedural memory. J Cogn Neurosci 1997;9:534.

3. Tucker MA, Hirota Y, Wamsley EJ, et al. A daytime nap containing solely non-REM sleep enhances declarative but not procedural memory. Neurobiol Learn Mem 2006;86:241.

4. Schabus M, Gruber G, Parapatics S, et al. Sleep spindles and their significance for declarative memory consolidation. Sleep 2004;27:1479.

5. Stickgold R, Whidbee D, Schirmer B, et al. Visual discrimination task improvement: a multi-step process occurring during sleep. J Cogn Neurosci 2000;12:246.

6. Walker MP, Brakefield T, Morgan A, et al. Practice with sleep makes perfect: sleep-dependent motor skill learning. Neuron 2002;35:205.

7. Huber R, Ghilardi MF, Massimini M, et al. Local sleep and learning. Nature 2004;430:78.

8. Wagner U, Gais S, Born J. Emotional memory formation is enhanced across sleep intervals with high amounts of rapid eye movement sleep. Learn Mem 2001;8:112.

9. Nishida M, Pearsall J, Buckner RL, et al. REM sleep, prefrontal theta, and the consolidation of human emotional memory. Cerebral Cortex 2009;19:1158.

10. Peigneux P, Laureys S, Fuchs S, et al. Are spatial memories strengthened in the human hippocampus during slow wave sleep? Neuron 2004;44:535.

11. Wamsley EJ, Tucker MA, Payne JD, et al. A brief nap is beneficial for human route-learning: the role of navigation experience and EEG spectral power. Learn Mem 2010;17:332.

12. Buzsaki G. Memory consolidation during sleep: a neurophysiological perspective. J Sleep Res 1998;7(Suppl 1):17.

13. Buzsaki G. Hippocampal sharp waves: their origin and significance. Brain Res 1986;398:242.

14. Dupret D, O'Neill J, Pleydell-Bouverie B, et al. The reorganization and reactivation of hippocampal maps predict spatial memory performance. Nat Neurosci 2010;13:995.

15. Tamminen J, Payne JD, Stickgold R, et al. Sleep spindle activity is associated with the integration of new memories and existing knowledge. J Neurosci 2010;30(43):14356–60.

16. Dumay N, Gaskell MG. Sleep-associated changes in the mental representation of spoken words. Psychol Sci 2007;18:35.

17. Payne JD, Schacter DL, Propper RE, et al. The role of sleep in false memory formation. Neurobiol Learn Mem 2009;92:327.

18. Wagner U, Gais S, Haider H, et al. Sleep inspires insight. Nature 2004;427:352.

19. Takashima A, Nieuwenhuis IL, Jensen O, et al. Shift from hippocampal to neocortical centered retrieval

network with consolidation. J Neurosci 2009;29:10087.

20. Takashima A, Petersson KM, Rutters F, et al. Declarative memory consolidation in humans: a prospective functional magnetic resonance imaging study. Proc Natl Acad Sci U S A 2006;103:756.

21. Payne JD, Kensinger EA. Sleep leads to changes in the emotional memory trace: evidence from fMRI. J Cogn Neurosci 2010. [Epub ahead of print]. DOI:10.1162/jocn.2010.21526.

22. Sterpenich V, Albouy G, Darsaud A, et al. Sleep promotes the neural reorganization of remote emotional memory. J Neurosci 2009;29:5143.

23. Frankland PW, Bontempi B. The organization of recent and remote memories. Nat Rev Neurosci 2005;6:119.

24. Baylor GW, Cavallero C. Memory sources associated with REM and NREM dream reports throughout the night: a new look at the data. Sleep 2001;24:165.

25. Smith MR, Antrobus JS, Gordon E, et al. Motivation and affect in REM sleep and the mentation reporting process. Conscious Cogn 2004;13:501.

26. Kudrimoti HS, Barnes CA, McNaughton BL. Reactivation of hippocampal cell assemblies: effects of behavioral state, experience, and EEG dynamics. J Neurosci 1999;19:4090.

27. Wilson MA, McNaughton BL. Reactivation of hippocampal ensemble memories during sleep. Science 1994;265:676.

28. Stickgold R, Malia A, Maguire D, et al. Replaying the game: hypnagogic images in normals and amnesics. Science 2000;290:350.

29. Wamsley EJ, Perry K, Djonlagic I, et al. Cognitive replay of visuomotor learning at sleep onset: temporal dynamics and relationship to task performance. Sleep 2010;33:59.

30. Ji D, Wilson MA. Coordinated memory replay in the visual cortex and hippocampus during sleep. Nat Neurosci 2007;10:100.

31. Nadasdy Z, Hirase H, Czurko A, et al. Replay and time compression of recurring spike sequences in the hippocampus. J Neurosci 1999;19:9497.

32. Fosse MJ, Fosse R, Hobson JA, et al. Dreaming and episodic memory: a functional dissociation? J Cogn Neurosci 2003;15:1.

33. Braun AR, Balkin TJ, Wesenten NJ, et al. Regional cerebral blood flow throughout the sleep-wake cycle. An H2(15)O PET study. Brain 1997;120:1173.

34. Hasselmo ME. Neuromodulation: acetylcholine and memory consolidation. Trends Cogn Sci 1999;3:351.

35. Plihal W, Born J. Memory consolidation in human sleep depends on inhibition of glucocorticoid release. Neuroreport 1999;10:2741.

36. Payne JD, Nadel L. Sleep, dreams, and memory consolidation: the role of the stress hormone cortisol. Learn Mem 2004;11:671.

37. Cai DJ, Mednick SA, Harrison EM, et al. REM, not incubation, improves creativity by priming associative networks. Proc Natl Acad Sci U S A 2009;106:10130.

38. Paller KA, Voss JL. Memory reactivation and consolidation during sleep. Learn Mem 2004;11:664.

39. Louie K, Wilson MA. Temporally structured replay of awake hippocampal ensemble activity during rapid eye movement sleep. Neuron 2001;29:145.

40. Walker MP, van der Helm E. Overnight therapy? The role of sleep in emotional brain processing. Psychol Bull 2009;135:731.

41. Freud S. The interpretation of dreams. New York: Random House; 1900.

42. Cartwright R. The relation of daytime events to the dreams that follow. In: Hartmann E, editor. Sleep and dreaming. Boston: Little, Brown and Company; 1970. p. 227.

43. Baekeland F. Laboratory studies of effects of presleep events on sleep and dreams. Int Psychiatry Clin 1970;7:49.

44. Breger L, Hunter I, Lane RW. The effect of stress on dreams, vol. 7. New York: International Universities Press; 1971.

45. Foulkes D, Rechtschaffen A. Presleep determinants of dream content: effect of two films. Percept Mot Skills 1964;19:983.

46. Goodenough DR, Witkin HA, Koulack D, et al. The effects of stress films on dream affect and on respiration and eye-movement activity during Rapid-Eye-Movement sleep. Psychophysiology 1975;12:313.

47. Witkin HA, Lewis HB. The relation of experimentally induced presleep experiences to dreams. A report on method and preliminary findings. J Am Psychoanal Assoc 1965;13:819.

48. Dement WC, Kahn E, Roffwarg HP. The influence of the laboratory situation on the dreams of the experimental subject. J Nerv Ment Dis 1965;140:119.

49. Nielsen TA, Kuiken D, Alain G, et al. Immediate and delayed incorporations of events into dreams: further replication and implications for dream function. J Sleep Res 2004;13:327.

50. Cavallero C. Dream sources, associative mechanisms, and temporal dimension. Sleep 1987;10:78.

51. Cavallero C, Foulkes D, Hollifield M, et al. Memory sources of REM and NREM dreams. Sleep 1990;13:449.

52. Hall C, Van de Castle R. The content analysis of dreams. New York: Appleton-Century-Crofts; 1966.

53. Hall C, Nordby V. The individual and his dreams. New York: New American Library; 1972.

54. Domhoff GW. The scientific study of dreams. Washington, DC: American Psychological Association; 2002.

55. Pivik T, Foulkes D. NREM mentation: relation to personality, orientation time, and time of night. J Consult Clin Psychol 1968;32:144.

56. Foulkes D. Nonrapid eye movement mentation. Exp Neurol 1967;(Suppl 4):28.

57. Wamsley EJ, Hirota Y, Tucker MA, et al. Circadian and ultradian influences on dreaming: a dual rhythm model. Brain Res Bull 2007;71:347.

58. Cavallero C, Cicogna P, Natale V, et al. Slow wave sleep dreaming. Sleep 1992;15:562.

59. Antrobus J. REM and NREM sleep reports: comparison of word frequencies by cognitive classes. Psychophysiology 1983;20:562.

60. Antrobus J, Kondo T, Reinsel R, et al. Dreaming in the late morning: summation of REM and diurnal cortical activation. Conscious Cogn 1995;4:275.

61. Verdone P. Temporal reference of manifest dream content. Percept Mot Skills 1965;20(Suppl):1253.

62. Baekeland F, Resch R, Katz D. Presleep mentation and dream reports. I. Cognitive style, contiguity to sleep, and time of night. Arch Gen Psychiatry 1968;19:300.

63. Natale V, Battaglia D. Temporal dating of autobiographical memories associated to REM and NREM dreams. Imagination, Cognition, and Personality 1990–91;10:279.

64. Grenier J, Cappeliez P, St-Onge M, et al. Temporal references in dreams and autobiographical memory. Mem Cognit 2005;33:280.

65. Nielsen TA, Powell RA. The 'dream-lag' effect: a 6-day temporal delay in dream content incorporation. Psychiatr J Univ Ott 1989;14:561.

66. Wamsley EJ, Tucker M, Payne JD, et al. Dreaming of a learning task is associated with enhanced sleep-dependent memory consolidation. Curr Biol 2010; 20:850.

67. Siegel JM. The REM sleep-memory consolidation hypothesis. Science 2001;294:1058.

68. Vertes RP. Memory consolidation in sleep: dream or reality. Neuron 2004;44:135.

69. McClelland JL, McNaughton BL, O'Reilly RC. Why there are complementary learning systems in the hippocampus and neocortex: insights from the successes and failures of connectionist models of learning and memory. Psychol Rev 1995;102:419.

70. Spreng RN, Grady CL. Patterns of brain activity supporting autobiographical memory, prospection, and theory of mind, and their relationship to the default mode network. J Cogn Neurosci 2010;22: 1112.

71. Schacter DL, Addis DR, Buckner RL. Remembering the past to imagine the future: the prospective brain. Nat Rev Neurosci 2007;8:657.

72. Winson J. The biology and function of rapid eye movement sleep. Curr Opin Neurobiol 1993;3:243.

73. Ficc H, Kramer F, Lichtman J. The mnemonic function of dreaming. Sleep Res 1977;6:122.

74. De Koninck J, Christ G, Hebert G, et al. Language learning efficiency, dreams and REM sleep. Psychiatr J Univ Ott 1990;15:91.

75. De Koninck J, Christ G, Rinfret N, et al. Dreams during language learning: when and how is the new language integrated. Psychiatr J Univ Ott 1988;13:72.

76. Cartwright R, Agargun MY, Kirkby J, et al. Relation of dreams to waking concerns. Psychiatry Res 2006; 141:261.

77. Lara-Carrasco J, Nielsen TA, Solomonova E, et al. Overnight emotional adaptation to negative stimuli is altered by REM sleep deprivation and is correlated with intervening dream emotions. J Sleep Res 2009;18:178.

78. De Koninck JM, Koulack D. Dream content and adaptation to a stressful situation. J Abnorm Psychol 1975;84:250.

The Neurocognitive Effects of Sleep Disruption in Children and Adolescents

Louise M. O'Brien, PhD[a,b,*]

KEYWORDS

- Behavior • Learning • School performance • Mood
- Sleep disorder

Disrupted sleep in children, whether attributable to poor sleep hygiene, sleep restriction, or an underlying sleep disorder, is associated with a wide range of behavioral, cognitive, and mood impairments. Sleep problems are common in children, with rates between 25% and 40%,[1] and are frequently underrecognized, even though most problems can be effectively treated. In the National Sleep Foundation's Sleep In America Poll,[2] approximately 70% of parents of young children surveyed reported that their child had at least one sleep problem a few nights per week, yet only a minority (<15%) reported this information to their pediatrician. Adolescence is associated with a natural delay in circadian rhythms, and so it is perhaps not surprising that more than half of adolescents reported feeling sleepy during the day,[3] although only 16% believed that they had a sleep problem. Interestingly, even fewer of the parents (7%) in the same poll believed that their adolescent had a sleep problem.

Disruption or fragmentation of sleep often manifests in children as hyperactivity, inattention, poor concentration, poor impulse control, disruptive behavior problems, emotional lability, and poor school performance. Adolescents may be more likely to exhibit poor concentration, depressive symptoms, and excessive daytime sleepiness than hyperactivity, the latter of which is more commonly observed in younger children. Furthermore, the poor sleep habits of young children also affect parents, who have been reported to lose an estimated 200 hours of sleep per year because of their children's sleep disruption.[2] It is important to note that most of what we know about the neurocognitive effects of sleep disruption in childhood is based largely on data from studies measuring associations and correlations rather than proven fact. Ongoing randomized controlled trials in this field will provide us with more robust evidence in the future. This article highlights current understanding of the daytime consequences of sleep disruption in children and adolescents.

CULTURAL

What constitutes normal sleep? Few large-scale epidemiological studies have been conducted to define normal sleep parameters in childhood, and in those studies that have attempted to investigate normal sleep, methodologies differ widely. Childhood and adolescence is a time of rapid growth and maturation; therefore, what is considered

This article originally appeared in the October 2009 issue of *Child and Adolescent Psychiatric Clinics of North America* 18:4.

[a] Sleep Disorders Center, Department of Neurology, University of Michigan, Med Inn Building Room C736, 1500 E. Medical Center Drive, Ann Arbor, MI 48109-5845, USA
[b] Department of Oral and Maxillofacial Surgery, University Hospital, Taubman Center, B1, 1500 East Medical Center Drive, University of Michigan, Ann Arbor, MI 48109–5018, USA
* Department of Neurology, Sleep Disorders Center, University of Michigan, Med Inn Building Room C736, 1500 East Medical Center Drive, Ann Arbor, MI 48109-5845.
E-mail address: louiseo@med.umich.edu

normal sleep is a dynamic and complex process. Normal sleep may be defined culturally in terms of what fits with societal or parental expectations, irrespective of the biology of sleep. How abnormal sleep is defined may depend on whether the sleep does not fit within these cultural boundaries, or it may also be defined in terms of associated daytime morbidities. There is wide variation in the biology of sleep, the societal and cultural expectations of normal sleep, the developmental and physical and emotional changes that occur, and the developmental changes in sleep across different stages in child development. Thus, it is operationally difficult to define what constitutes problematic sleep.

POOR SLEEP HYGIENE/INSUFFICIENT SLEEP

We are a 24-hour society. Many young children and adolescents do not obtain enough sleep for a variety of reasons, including family schedules, chaotic living arrangements, television/computer/cell phone use in the bedroom after designated bedtimes, and after-school activities. There are often not enough hours in the day to accomplish what is wanted, and all too often it is sleep that is compromised. Data from the Zurich Longitudinal Studies,[4] which followed Swiss children from infancy to adolescence, provided percentile curves for sleep duration across the pediatric age range. Total sleep time decreased from approximately 14 hours in infancy, to 11 hours in school-aged children, to 8 hours in adolescence. More recently, the National Sleep Foundation Poll of children in the United States found that the average duration of time school-aged children spend sleeping is approximately 8 to 9 hours,[2] which is less than the 10 to 11 hours recommended by the American

Academy of Sleep Medicine.[5] Despite this fact, few large-scale studies have systematically investigated the impact of inadequate sleep on children. Clinically, however, there are many observations of the consequences of poor sleep, including inattention, externalizing behaviors, poor emotional control, and daytime sleepiness. **Table 1** summarizes the main daytime effects of sleep disruptions from several sleep disorders.

When assessing sleep objectively using actigraphy, sleep disruption has been associated with deficits in complex neurobehavioral tasks, such as selective attention in otherwise healthy children,[6] with the strength of the association being higher in younger children. In adolescents, shortened sleep time and irregular sleep schedules (poor sleep hygiene) are associated with impaired school performance, as reflected by lower grades.[7]

Few studies of sleep deprivation have been conducted in children. However, data from adults, including functional neuroimaging studies, provide substantial evidence that sleep deprivation negatively impacts vigilance, cognitive performance, and learning.[8,9] Acute sleep restriction of 1 night in children is associated with an increase in behaviors such as yawning and daydreaming, as well as inattentive behaviors, although this study did not find an increase in hyperactivity or impulsivity.[10] Partial sleep restriction studies in children have shown that even after restricting sleep to 6.5 hours (third graders and above) or 8.0 hours (first and second graders) as compared with the control duration of 10.0 hours per night for 3 weeks, those with restricted sleep were more likely to have academic problems and attention problems.[11] Again, no increase in hyperactive behaviors was observed in this teacher-report study.

Table 1
Daytime effects of sleep disorders

	Hyperactivity/ Impulsivity	Inattention	ADHD Symptoms	Aggression/ Conduct Problems	Poor School Performance	Depression/ Anxiety
Poor sleep hygiene	√	√	√	√	√	√
Sleep restriction	√	√	√	√	√	√
Circadian rhythm problems	—	√	√	—	√	√
SDB	√	√	√	√	√	√
RLS/PLM	√	√	√	√	—	√
Narcolepsy	—	√	√	—	√	√
Insomnia	—	√	√	√	√	√

Abbreviations: √, published literature supports association; —, no published data; ADHD, attention-deficit hyperactivity disorder; RLS/PLM, restless legs syndrome/periodic limb movement; SDB, sleep-disordered breathing.

In a longitudinal study of sixth, seventh, and eighth graders, those with shorter sleep durations were more likely to have reduced self-esteem, poor grades, and an increase in depressive symptoms.[12]

DELAYED SLEEP PHASE SYNDROME

Circadian rhythms develop throughout life and are entwined with the light-dark cycle. Optimal sleep occurs when the internal circadian cycle is aligned with the external sleep-wake schedule, and when this alignment becomes destabilized, circadian rhythm sleep disorders can occur. One of the most relevant circadian disorders in childhood and adolescence is delayed sleep phase disorder, where the sleep period is delayed in relation to the required or desired sleep-wake times. As children develop and reach puberty, there is a natural tendency to fall asleep later with greater difficulty waking up early. The circadian cycle undergoes changes during adolescence, and a phase preference for eveningness (owl), as opposed to morningness (lark), has been reported to be associated with pubertal development.[13] Delayed sleep phase syndrome may be an extreme variant of these developmental shifts. It is no surprise to parents that as children get older they go to bed later and, coupled with early school start times, most adolescents have great difficultly waking on school mornings. Indeed, the National Sleep Foundation Poll reported that 70% of adolescents needed someone to wake them on school mornings.[3]

Common comorbidities of delayed sleep phase syndrome are attention-deficit hyperactivity disorder (ADHD)-like behaviors and depressive symptoms. Many children who are unable to fall asleep at the required time have daytime sleepiness at school, which may preclude full participation in classroom activities. Giannotti and colleagues[14] have shown that children with delayed sleep phase syndrome frequently have problems with daytime sleepiness, attention, emotional outbursts, and poor school achievement. In addition, they reported an increased frequency of physical injuries. Several studies have reported an association with ADHD, as well as oppositional problems and conduct disorder (for a review see Cardinali[15]). Mood disorders, particularly depression, are frequently associated with circadian rhythm problems. It can be a challenge for the clinician to treat these patients, as the relationships with behavioral or emotional problems are likely bidirectional with the circadian disorder.[16] Many of the adolescents with delayed sleep phase disorder are labeled as having behavioral problems, but if they are allowed to sleep until later in the morning, their symptoms abate.[17]

This finding raises the issue of school start times. The biological delay in the circadian system of adolescents coupled with early school start times has been associated with impaired school performance. Most of this work has been conducted in middle school and high school students, and several studies suggest that more time in bed is related to better school grades.[7] In a group of 800 Israeli preadolescents, investigators compared children who started school before 7:15 AM with those who started at 8:00 AM. They found that those who started earlier were more likely to complain of daytime sleepiness, doze off in class, and have more attention and concentration problems.[18] In a large survey of more than 3000 students, those reporting B grades or better were significantly more likely to go to bed between 10 and 50 minutes earlier and obtain 17 to 33 minutes more sleep than their peers who obtained C grades or below.[19] In a landmark study[20] that was the first large-scale longitudinal study of the effects of delayed school start times on the academic performance of children, 18,000 children were followed from 2 years before until 3 years after their schools delayed start times from 7:15 AM to 8:40 AM. Multiple improvements were observed from decreases in tardiness, increases in graduation rates, improved academic performance, and higher morale. These findings underscore the serious impact of early school start times on children's and adolescent's school performance, yet most schools still have start times that are not conducive to good performance (for a review see O'Malley and O'Malley[21]).

SLEEP-DISORDERED BREATHING

The cognitive and behavioral manifestations of sleep disruption are probably most well studied in children with sleep-disordered breathing (SDB). SDB describes a spectrum of sleep-related breathing problems ranging from snoring to obstructive sleep apnea and is most common in young school-aged children. Although there has been a considerable research effort in this area in the past few decades, the first reports of learning and behavioral problems in children with SDB were published in the late 1800s.[22] Behavioral dysregulation is the most commonly encountered comorbidity of SDB, and the vast majority of studies consistently report some association between SDB symptoms, or objective measures of SDB, and hyperactivity, impulsivity, and ADHD-like symptoms.[23–26] In a survey of more than 800 families using validated instruments,[23] symptoms of SDB were associated with hyperactive behaviors with a trend toward a dose-response relationship between reported snoring frequency and behavior.

Even in children with primary snoring (snoring in the absence of obstructive apneas), behavioral problems have been reported.[27] Children with SDB have been reported to have more inattention than other children, although the strength of the associations is not as robust as for hyperactivity. Continuous Performance Tests that can differentiate between types of attention, such as selective or sustained attention, show that children with SDB, even if only mild, exhibit deficits in attention when compared with control children.[28–30]

SBD and ADHD

The major features of ADHD (eg, inattention, hyperactivity, and impulsivity) are frequent manifestations of childhood SDB, and, thus, the relationship between these two disorders is of great interest. Parental reports of children with ADHD show that these children demonstrate a number of sleep problems, with a frequency five times greater than that of otherwise healthy children.[31] Children with ADHD are more likely to snore than their peers, with some studies suggesting that snoring is more common in those with the hyperactive/impulsive subtype of ADHD.[32] Polysomnographic data are less clear in terms of an association between SDB and ADHD, with many studies failing to find a consistent relationship. However, recent data, including a systematic review,[33] suggest that children with ADHD are indeed more likely to have SDB, albeit rather mild in severity. In a study of school-aged children undergoing polysomnography before removal of enlarged tonsils and adenoids (typically for SDB), formal diagnoses of ADHD were found in almost a third of children,[29] yet half of these children did not fulfill criteria for a diagnosis of ADHD a year after adenotonsillectomy. Disturbances of prefrontal cortex functions have been implicated in deficits observed in children with ADHD,[34] as the prefrontal cortex is believed to play a critical role in the regulation of arousal, sleep, and attention.[35]

Conduct Disorder and Aggressive Behaviors

Conduct problems and aggressive behaviors are beginning to receive more attention in the SDB literature. These behaviors pose a particular problem for schools, which often have local, state, and national programs to address this public health issue. Although studies are more limited than those of hyperactivity and inattention, several large survey investigations have found a relationship between parentally reported symptoms of SDB and aggressive behaviors.[24,26,36] Based on the reports of parents surveyed at a general pediatric clinic, children between 2 and 14 years old at high risk for SDB, as identified by a validated screening tool, were 2 to 3 times more likely to be bullying, constantly fighting, quarrelsome, and cruel in comparison with other children.[36] Conduct problems are associated with a myriad of well-studied social and cultural underpinnings, although it is possible that SDB or other reasons for sleep disruption may contribute to some of these behaviors. Children with aggressive behaviors have also been found to have electroencephalogram slowing during wakefulness,[37] which may reflect deficient levels of arousal or excessive daytime sleepiness, likely mediated via the prefrontal cortex.[38]

Cognitive Dysfunction

As well as behavioral manifestations, there are many reports of children with SDB demonstrating cognitive impairments, although the findings of such studies are not as robust as those for behavioral dysregulation. Reduced intelligence, as measured by either full-scale intelligence quotient (IQ) or subscale IQ (eg, verbal IQ), has been reported.[28,39,40] However, most studies still report IQ scores within normal limits, the differences being perhaps explained by control children frequently scoring higher than would be anticipated. Memory deficits also have been reported,[41,42] although this finding is not universal even in large samples with variable degrees of SDB severity. Differences in aspects of memory measured across studies (eg, declarative memory, verbal memory, or working memory) may have contributed to these discrepancies.

Attention and working memory have a close relationship with executive functioning, which is involved in the ability to plan, develop, and carry out problem solving and is critical for normal psychological development. Impairments in executive functioning have been commonly reported in adults with SDB[43] and more recently in children,[25,40] including preschoolers.[44] Executive functioning is a complex domain to measure because it is difficult to isolate from other cognitive abilities. Furthermore, deficits in executive functioning may alter recruitment of other cognitive abilities, which may negatively impact behavior. The prefrontal cortex has been implicated in executive dysfunction observed in SDB (see Beebe and Gozal[45]). Children who perform poorly at school are more likely to have SDB, and a seminal study showed that a six- to ninefold increase in sleep-associated gas exchange abnormalities was evident in first-grade children who were performing at the bottom 10th percentile of their class.[46] Even reports of frequent snoring (in the absence of hypoxemia) have been associated with twice the risk of poor performance in mathematics and spelling, a relationship that appears to have a dose-response effect.[47]

The impact of SDB on behavior and cognition may be age dependent. Younger children may be more vulnerable to cognitive deficits, and most studies reporting an association were conducted in preschool or early school-aged children. Even snoring infants perform worse on the Mental Development Index of the Bayley Scales of Infant Development than nonsnoring infants.[48] Older children tend to show weaker associations,[25,41] possibly suggesting a window of vulnerability in the developing brain. (The reader is referred to Beebe[49] for an excellent review on the impact of pediatric SDB on behavior and cognition.)

When discussing neurobehavioral manifestations of sleep disturbance, most research, and therefore most of the focus, is on SDB. However, neurobehavioral deficits have also been observed in children with other sleep disorders,[50] several of which will be discussed in the following sections.

RESTLESS LEGS SYNDROME/PERIODIC LIMB MOVEMENTS

Hyperactivity is most commonly associated with SDB. Nonetheless, restless legs syndrome (RLS) and periodic limb movements (PLM) during sleep in children are also strongly associated with hyperactivity.[51,52] Children and adolescents with PLMs have a high frequency of ADHD,[53,54] and conversely children with ADHD are more likely to have PLMs during sleep.[55] One possibility is that RLS and PLMs may fragment sleep and lead to daytime sleepiness and symptoms similar to ADHD. Strong independent interrelationships between children with RLS/PLMs and symptoms of ADHD have been found,[56] and such relationships may even be stronger than those between SDB and ADHD.[57] There is also evidence to suggest that children with RLS may be at increased risk for depression and anxiety.[58]

Both RLS and PLMs respond to dopaminergic therapy. Interestingly, Walters and colleagues[52] found that dopaminergic therapy was associated with improved behavior, with three of seven children with ADHD no longer qualifying for a diagnosis of ADHD. Iron is also essential for the metabolism of dopamine, and both PLMs and ADHD have been associated with reduced levels of ferritin.[59,60] Supplementation with iron has been shown to successfully treat PLMs in children,[59] and although there is a case report of improved behavior in a child with ADHD when treated with iron supplementation,[61] there are no studies that have investigated the role of iron in ADHD. As the mechanisms that link PLMs and behavioral problems

have not been fully delineated, explanations for the behavioral improvement could include restoration of consolidated sleep or a common dopaminergic deficit shared by PLMs and ADHD.

NARCOLEPSY

Narcolepsy is rare in preschoolers and uncommon in young children. Affected school-aged children have been reported to have impaired concentration, poor school performance, executive dysfunction, and emotional instability. There are reports of children with narcolepsy being described as lazy and more likely to have negative peer interactions, which can feed the cycle of negative behavior and schooling problems. Depressive symptoms, as well as inattention and ADHD-like behaviors, have been reported in children with narcolepsy, although most information regarding daytime manifestations is obtained from clinical reports. One study of 42 children with narcolepsy and a group of "sleepy children" as controls[62] found a range of psychosocial problems, including depression. Both narcoleptic children and sleepy controls had higher rates of depression, increased behavioral problems, and impaired quality of life than would be expected from a healthy control group. These findings suggest that the daytime sleepiness associated with narcolepsy may be driving the daytime psychiatric impairments. In adolescents and adults with narcolepsy, there are frequent histories consistent with behavioral problems as children, including many being labeled with ADHD-like behaviors.

TREATMENT OF SLEEP PROBLEMS

Although it is beyond the scope of this article to discuss treatment options, it is noteworthy to mention that treatment of sleep disruptions, whether caused by insufficient sleep, poor sleep hygiene, SDB, RLS, or circadian problems, can improve daytime functioning. For example, the most well-studied disorder in terms of its impact on neurobehavioral function is SDB. Multiple studies have shown that treatment of childhood SDB by adenotonsillectomy improves both behavior and cognition.[29,30,46,63] In one study of children undergoing adenotonsillectomy,[29] 22 of 78 children had a formal diagnosis of ADHD before surgery, yet 50% of these children no longer qualified for a diagnosis 1 year after surgery. In children with poor school performance who underwent surgery for SDB, school grades were significantly improved the year following surgery in comparison with those who also had SDB but whose parents elected not to seek treatment.[46] Quality of life is also improved when children with SDB are treated with adenotonsillectomy.[64]

Treatments of other sleep disorders have been less well studied in terms of behavioral outcomes than has SDB. However, there are case reports and anecdotal evidence of improved behaviors, such as ADHD symptoms, aggression, defiance, and moodiness, when children receive treatment for RLS/PLMs.[65] Similarly, improved behavior, mood, and less stressful family dynamics have all been reported following treatment for circadian rhythm disorders. As already described, readjusting school start times to better align with biological sleep-wake rhythms is associated with improvement in school performance, social interactions, behavior, and emotional outbursts. In parallel with treatment of specific sleep problems, addressing problematic sleep hygiene by both parent and child education is also vitally important. Improvement in sleep hygiene and ensuring children and adolescents receive sufficient time for sleep decreases daytime sleepiness and is associated with improved daytime functioning both academically and socially.

IS THERE A COMMON THREAD?

The behavioral problems observed in multiple sleep disorders described in the preceding sections are remarkably similar: hyperactivity, inattention, conduct problems, depression, and cognitive/schooling problems. The vast majority of sleep disorders previously described, including SDB, result in fragmented sleep and daytime sleepiness. Thus, it is possible that the common feature of daytime sleepiness could play a role in the daytime morbidities. Children who are sleepy, whether as a result of ADHD, SDB, RLS, narcolepsy, or poor sleep hygiene, may have strong drives to stay awake, and as such develop hyperactive, stimulus-seeking behavior. Insufficient or inadequate sleep may, through induction of sleepiness, impair executive functioning, regulation of impulsivity, and control of emotions.[35] Improvement in sleep, whether by treatment of specific sleep disorders or by better sleep hygiene, is associated with less daytime sleepiness and subsequent reductions in problematic behavior. It is tempting to blame sleepiness as the common factor responsible for the resultant daytime deficits observed in a wide range of sleep disorders. However, as Beebe points out in his review,[49] while daytime sleepiness and neurobehavioral deficits may share a common cause, such as sleep disruption, one should be careful not to solely attribute impaired daytime function to sleepiness until there is clear evidence of physiological mechanisms by which these occur in childhood.

SUMMARY

Sleep disruption in childhood and adolescence is common and associated with multiple behavioral and cognitive impairments. It is important to note that many of the sleep problems discussed here may not occur in isolation. Similarly, there are bidirectional relationships with some sleep problems and psychiatric disorders, and it can sometimes be challenging to disentangle these often complex relationships. Childhood sleep problems are a significant source of stress for the whole family, as parental sleep is also affected, leading to a reduction in the level of effective parenting. Yet many parents are unaware of the major impact of sleep disruption on their child's learning and behavior. Given the impact of sleep disruptions on learning and behavior, sleep education about the broad meaning of "normal" sleep, the impact of sleep disruption on daytime functioning, and how good sleep hygiene and treatment for specific disorders can significantly improve well-being is warranted.

REFERENCES

1. Owens J. Epidemiology of sleep disorders during childhood. In: Sheldon S, Ferber R, Kryger MH, editors. Principles and practices of pediatric sleep medicine. Philadelphia: Elsevier Saunders; 2005. p. 27–33.
2. National Sleep Foundation. Sleep in America poll: sleep and children. 2008. Available at: http://www.sleepfoundation.org/site/c.huIXKjM0IxF/b.2419041/k.1302/2004_Sleep_in_America_Poll.htm. Accessed December 17, 2008.
3. National Sleep Foundation. Sleep in America poll: American's sleepy teens. 2008. Available at: http://www.sleepfoundation.org/site/c.huIXKjM0IxF/b.2419037/. Accessed December 17, 2008.
4. Iglowstein I, Jenni OG, Molinari L, et al. Sleep duration from infancy to adolescence: reference values and generational trends. Pediatrics 2003;111(2):302–7.
5. American Academy of Sleep Medicine. Web site. Available at: www.aasmnet.org. Accessed December 28, 2008.
6. Sadeh A, Gruber R, Raviv A. Sleep, neurobehavioral functioning, and behavior problems in school-age children. Child Dev 2002;73(2):405–17.
7. Wolfson AR, Carskadon MA. Understanding adolescents' sleep patterns and school performance: a critical appraisal. Sleep Med Rev 2003;7(6):491–506.
8. Lim J, Dinges DF. Sleep deprivation and vigilant attention. Ann N Y Acad Sci 2008;1129:305–22.

9. Chee MW, Chuah LY. Functional neuroimaging insights into how sleep and sleep deprivation affect memory and cognition. Curr Opin Neurol 2008; 21(4):417–23.

10. Fallone G, Acebo C, Arnett JT, et al. Effects of acute sleep restriction on behavior, sustained attention, and response inhibition in children. Percept Mot Skills 2001;93(1):213–29.

11. Fallone G, Acebo C, Seifer R, et al. Experimental restriction of sleep opportunity in children: effects on teacher ratings. Sleep 2005;28(12):1561–7.

12. Fredriksen K, Rhodes J, Reddy R, et al. Sleepless in Chicago: tracking the effects of adolescent sleep loss during the middle school years. Child Dev 2004;75(1):84–95.

13. Carskadon MA, Vieira C, Acebo C. Association between puberty and delayed phase preference. Sleep 1993;16(3):258–62.

14. Giannotti F, Cortesi F, Sebastiani T, et al. Circadian preference, sleep and daytime behaviour in adolescence. J Sleep Res 2002;11(3):191–9.

15. Cardinali D. The human body circadian: how the biological clock influences sleep and emotion. Neuro Endocrinol Lett 2000;21:9–15.

16. Dahl R, Lewin DS. Pathways to adolescent health sleep regulation and behavior. J Adolesc Health 2002;31(6):175–84.

17. Millman RP. Excessive sleepiness in adolescents and young adults: causes, consequences, and treatment strategies. Pediatrics 2005;115(6): 1774–86.

18. Epstein R, Chillag N, Lavie P. Starting times of school: effects on daytime functioning of fifth-grade children in Israel. Sleep 1998;21(3):250–6.

19. Wolfson AR, Carskadon MA. Sleep schedules and daytime functioning in adolescents. Child Dev 1998;69(4):875–87.

20. Wahlstrom K. Changing times: findings from the first longitudinal study of later high school start times. NASSP Bulletin 2002;86(633):3–21.

21. O'Malley EB, O'Malley MB. School start time and its impact on learning and behavior. In: Ivanenko A, editor. Sleep and psychiatric disorders in children and adolescents. New York: Informa Healthcare; 2008. p. 79–94.

22. Hill W. On some causes of backwardness and stupidity in children. BMJ 1889;1:711–2.

23. Chervin RD, Archbold KH, Dillon JE, et al. Inattention, hyperactivity, and symptoms of sleep-disordered breathing. Pediatrics 2002;109(3):449–56.

24. Gottlieb DJ, Vezina RM, Chase C, et al. Symptoms of sleep-disordered breathing in 5-year-old children are associated with sleepiness and problem behaviors. Pediatrics 2003;112(4):870–7.

25. Beebe DW, Wells CT, Jeffries J, et al. Neuropsychological effects of pediatric obstructive sleep apnea. J Int Neuropsychol Soc 2004;10(7):962–75.

26. Rosen CL, Storfer-Isser A, Taylor HG, et al. Increased behavioral morbidity in school-aged children with sleep-disordered breathing. Pediatrics 2004;114(6):1640–8.

27. O'Brien LM, Mervis CB, Holbrook CR, et al. Neurobehavioral implications of habitual snoring in children. Pediatrics 2004;114(1):44–9.

28. Blunden S, Lushington K, Kennedy D, et al. Behavior and neurocognitive performance in children aged 5-10 years who snore compared to controls. J Clin Exp Neuropsychol 2000;22(5):554–68.

29. Chervin RD, Ruzicka DL, Giordani BJ, et al. Sleep-disordered breathing, behavior, and cognition in children before and after adenotonsillectomy. Pediatrics 2006;117(4):e769–78.

30. Galland BC, Dawes PJ, Tripp EG, et al. Changes in behavior and attentional capacity after adenotonsillectomy. Pediatr Res 2006;59(5):711–6.

31. Corkum P, Tannock R, Moldofsky H. Sleep disturbances in children with attention-deficit/hyperactivity disorder. J Am Acad Child Adolesc Psychiatry 1998;37(6):637–46.

32. LeBourgeois MK, Avis K, Mixon M, et al. Snoring, sleep quality, and sleepiness across attention-deficit/hyperactivity disorder subtypes. Sleep 2004; 27(3):520–5.

33. Cortese S, Konofal E, Yateman N, et al. Sleep and alertness in children with attention-deficit/hyperactivity disorder: a systematic review of the literature. Sleep 2006;29(4):504–11.

34. Barkley R. Attention-deficit/hyperactivity disorder, self-regulation, and time: toward a more comprehensive theory. J Dev Behav Pediatr 1997;18(4):271–9.

35. Dahl RE. The impact of inadequate sleep on children's daytime cognitive function. Semin Pediatr Neurol 1996;3(1):44–50.

36. Chervin RD, Dillon JE, Archbold KH, et al. Conduct problems and symptoms of sleep disorders in children. J Am Acad Child Adolesc Psychiatry 2003; 42(2):201–8.

37. Forssman H, Frey TS. Electroencephalograms of boys with behavior disorders. Acta Psychiatr Neurol Scand 1953;28:61–73.

38. Thomas M, Sing H, Belenky G, et al. Neural basis of alertness and cognitive performance impairments during sleepiness. I. Effects of 24 h of sleep deprivation on waking human regional brain activity. J Sleep Res 2000;9(4):335–52.

39. O'Brien LM, Mervis CB, Holbrook CR, et al. Neurobehavioral correlates of sleep-disordered breathing in children. J Sleep Res 2004;13(2):165–72.

40. Gottlieb DJ, Chase C, Vezina RM, et al. Sleep-disordered breathing symptoms are associated with poorer cognitive function in 5-year-old children. J Pediatr 2004;145(4):458–64.

41. Kaemingk KL, Pasvogel AE, Goodwin JL, et al. Learning in children and sleep disordered

breathing: findings of the Tucson Children's Assessment of Sleep Apnea (tuCASA) prospective cohort study. J Int Neuropsychol Soc 2003;9(7):1016–26.

42. Kennedy JD, Blunden S, Hirte C, et al. Reduced neurocognition in children who snore. Pediatr Pulmonol 2004;37(4):330–7.

43. Saunamäki T, Jehkonen M. A review of executive functions in obstructive sleep apnea syndrome. Acta Neurol Scand 2007;115(1):1–11.

44. Karpinski AC, Scullin MH, Montgomery-Downs HE. Risk for sleep-disordered breathing and executive function in preschoolers. Sleep Med 2008;9(4):418–24.

45. Beebe DW, Gozal D. Obstructive sleep apnea and the prefrontal cortex: towards a comprehensive model linking nocturnal upper airway obstruction to daytime cognitive and behavioral deficits. J Sleep Res 2002;11(1):1–16.

46. Gozal D. Sleep-disordered breathing and school performance in children. Pediatrics 1998;102(3 Pt 1):616–20.

47. Urschitz MS, Guenther A, Eggebrecht E, et al. Snoring, intermittent hypoxia and academic performance in primary school children. Am J Respir Crit Care Med 2003;168(4):464–8.

48. Montgomery-Downs HE, Gozal D. Snore-associated sleep fragmentation in infancy: mental development effects and contribution of secondhand cigarette smoke exposure. Pediatrics 2006;117(3):e496–502.

49. Beebe DW. Neurobehavioral morbidity associated with disordered breathing during sleep in children: a comprehensive review. Sleep 2006;29(9):1115–34.

50. Blunden SL, Beebe DW. The contribution of intermittent hypoxia, sleep debt and sleep disruption to daytime performance deficits in children: consideration of respiratory and non-respiratory sleep disorders. Sleep Med Rev 2006;10(2):109–18.

51. Chervin RD, Archbold KH, Dillon JE, et al. Associations between symptoms of inattention, hyperactivity, restless legs, and periodic leg movements. Sleep 2002;25(2):213–8.

52. Walters AS, Mandelbaum DE, Lewin DS, et al. Dopaminergic therapy in children with restless legs/periodic limb movements in sleep and ADHD. Dopaminergic Therapy Study Group. Pediatr Neurol 2000;22(3):182–6.

53. Picchietti DL, Walters AS. Moderate to severe periodic limb movement disorder in childhood and adolescence. Sleep 1999;22(3):297–300.

54. Corkum P, Tannock R, Moldofsky H, et al. Actigraphy and parental ratings of sleep in children with attention-deficit/hyperactivity disorder (ADHD). Sleep 2001;24(3):303–12.

55. Picchietti DL, Underwood DJ, Farris WA, et al. Further studies on periodic limb movement disorder and restless legs syndrome in children with attention-deficit hyperactivity disorder. Mov Disord 1999;14(6):1000–7.

56. Cortese S, Konofal E, Lecendreux M, et al. Restless legs syndrome and attention-deficit/hyperactivity disorder: a review of the literature. Sleep 2005;28(8):1007–13.

57. Gaultney JF, Terrell DF, Gingras JL. Parent-reported periodic limb movement, sleep disordered breathing, bedtime resistance behaviors, and ADHD. Behav Sleep Med 2005;3(1):32–43.

58. Picchietti MA, Picchietti DL. Restless legs syndrome and periodic limb movement disorder in children and adolescents. Semin Pediatr Neurol 2008;15(2):91–9.

59. Simakajornboon N. Periodic limb movement disorder in children. Paediatr Respir Rev 2006;7(Suppl 1):S55–7.

60. Cortese S, Konofal E, Bernardina BD, et al. Sleep disturbances and serum ferritin levels in children with attention-deficit/hyperactivity disorder. Eur Child Adolesc Psychiatry 2009;18(7):393–9.

61. Konofal E, Cortese S, Lecendreux M, et al. Effectiveness of iron supplementation in a young child with attention-deficit/hyperactivity disorder. Pediatrics 2005;116(5):e732–4.

62. Stores G, Montgomery P, Wiggs L. The psychosocial problems of children with narcolepsy and those with excessive daytime sleepiness of uncertain origin. Pediatrics 2006;118(4):e1116–23.

63. Friedman BC, Hendeles-Amitai A, Kozminsky E, et al. Adenotonsillectomy improves neurocognitive function in children with obstructive sleep apnea syndrome. Sleep 2003;26(8):999–1005.

64. Mitchell RB, Kelly J. Outcomes and quality of life following adenotonsillectomy for sleep-disordered breathing in children. ORL J Otorhinolaryngol Relat Spec 2007;69(6):345–8.

65. Gingras JL, Gaultney JF. Restless legs syndrome and periodic limb movement disorders: association with ADHD. In: Ivanenko A, editor. Sleep and psychiatric disorders in children and adolescents. New York: Informa Healthcare; 2008. p. 193–224.

Sleepy Driving

Nelson B. Powell, MD, DDS[a,b,*],
Jason K.M. Chau, MD, MPH, FRCS(C)[c]

KEYWORDS

- Sleepiness • Drowsiness • Alcohol • Driving • Accidents
- Sleep apnea

SLEEPINESS AND DRIVING: A BRIEF REVIEW

Although the exact neurophysiologic mechanisms of sleep remain to be elucidated, there is ample scientific evidence identifying that adequate sleep is essential for healthy daily functioning and general well being.[1] Insufficient sleep may cause decrements in health and quality of life. Acute and chronic sleepiness is pervasive in our society and is generally the result of volitional insufficient sleep (sleep dept), or is secondary to an underlying sleep disorder such as obstructive sleep apnea (OSA) syndrome, narcolepsy, or insomnia.[2–6]

Regardless of the causes of sleepiness, driving while drowsy, tired, sleepy, or fatigued can result in human-error–related accidents and injuries due to decrements in neurobehavioral functions. These decrements may negatively affect reaction times and vigilance to such a degree to cause a motor vehicle accident.[7] Due to the large number of drivers on the United States highways, human-error accidents caused by sleepiness are of grave concern for public health and safety.[8–13] The National Transportation Safety Board (NTSB) reported in 2004 that there were 291 million individuals in the United States. Approximately 191 million were licensed to drive and of these about 42,000 die yearly in traffic-related accidents.[14] The National Sleep Foundation (NSF) "Sleep in America Poll" found that 51% of adult drivers polled admitted to driving drowsy and 17% reported falling asleep at the wheel in the previous year.[15] The prevalence of sleepiness in our society has been reported to be as high as 33%.[3,16] Hence, there is an immense pool of sleepy driving subjects, many of whom ignore or are oblivious to the signs of sleepiness and continue to drive. Some of the most common unambiguous behavioral signs of sleepy driving are: single or repetitive head drops (called microsleeps = lapses of ≥500 ms), heavy eyelids with frequent eye closures, and yawning. These signs are often ignored by the driver and as a result a sleepy accident could occur. It has been reported that subjects who fell asleep while driving usually knew they were experiencing fitful levels of sleepiness beforehand.[17] However, sleepy drivers are generally unable to predict when their sleep impairment has escalated to a point where sleep will overtake them without notice.[18] Unfortunately, at present there is no objective method to evaluate an unfit driver due to sleepiness alone.

BRIEF HISTORY OF SLEEPINESS

The peer-review literature is replete with years of data collection on the dangers of sleepy driving.[19–21] Many of these investigations suggest countermeasures and educational programs for drivers.[22–24] This approach has merit, but has not been widely implemented and unfortunately sleepy driving behavior still persists at high levels.[15] Hundreds of government and medical investigations concerning sleepiness and driving have

The authors have no financial disclosures or conflicts of interest with any person or company to report.
This article originally appeared in *Medical Clinics of North America* 94:3.
[a] Department of Otolaryngology Head and Neck Surgery, Stanford University School of Medicine, Palo Alto, Stanford, CA 94305, USA
[b] Department of Psychiatry and Behavioral Science, Stanford University Sleep and Research Center, Stanford University School of Medicine, Palo Alto, Stanford, CA 94305, USA
[c] Department of Otolaryngology-Head and Neck Surgery, University of Manitoba, GB421 820 Sherbrook Street, Winnipeg, Manitoba R3A 1R9, Canada
* Corresponding author. 750 Welch Road, Suite 317, Palo Alto, CA 94304.
E-mail address: nelsonpowell@sbcglobal.net

Sleep Med Clin 6 (2011) 117–124
doi:10.1016/j.jsmc.2010.12.006

been published, yet they have either not reached the public and health care providers or they have not been given adequate attention. Therefore, a disconnect exists between the published information available and the level of understanding among the population as a whole. In fact the public's understanding of sleep in general lags far behind the advances reported in the scientific literature. This gap needs to be improved.

What Was Previously Accomplished?

To emphasize that much has been uncovered about sleepiness, a literature search of Medline (PubMed) and Ovid databases was conducted. Key words used in the search strategy included: drowsiness, sleepiness and accidents, drowsiness and accidents, drowsiness and driving, sleepiness and driving. Non-English articles that had an abstract in English were included in the overall number count. Peer-reviewed articles dating from the early 1920s (Ovid) through the present day were included in the survey (PubMed goes back only to 1950) (**Fig. 1**). Two early examples are presented so the reader can fully appreciate that investigations of sleepiness have been around for many years. In 1921, McComas[25] reported on the effect of altitude on a subject flying in an airplane at up to 20,000 feet. Although not a driving experience per se, he examined lowered oxygen tensions as related to human motor mechanism activity, impaired vision, early fatigue, and coordination disturbances. The subject underwent 50 tests each at 4 different altitudes. The outcomes suggested that there were alterations of higher brain functions along with drowsiness and irritability. In 1938 Mayer[26] reported on the human factor in the prevention of (French) traffic accidents. He noted in part that 77% of traffic accidents were due to psychological factors secondary to a lack of attention, fatigue, drowsiness, and/or imprudence.

What Have We Now Accomplished?

An excellent review article by Ellen and colleagues[27] reported on motor vehicle crash risks in sleep apnea. The objective was to determine if drivers with sleep apnea have an increased risk of motor vehicle accidents and if sleep apnea severity and excessive daytime sleepiness (EDS) could affect driving risks. Forty-one evidence-based medicine studies of noncommercial drivers with sleep apnea were identified. A 2- to 3-times greater crash rate was identified in this group at a statistically significant level. Commercial drivers had comparatively smaller crash rates. Approximately 50% of the studies included in the review showed an increased risk for crashes with increased OSA severity, whereas the remaining

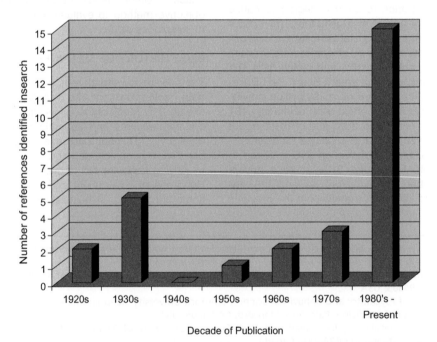

Decade of Publication

Fig. 1. November 2009 search results of Ovid and PubMed databases using the key words "drowsiness," "sleepiness," "drowsiness AND accidents," "sleepiness AND accidents," "drowsiness AND driving," and "sleepiness AND driving." The numbers of articles identified for a given decade are given on the Y-axis and their decade of publication on the X-axis. After 1980, more than 10,000 references were identified.

50% did not show this finding. Treatment of OSA was consistent with improvement of driver performance across all studies.

The Problem

Contrast the early research above to the current standards below and, although there is more sophisticated methodology today, the goals remain very similar. Sleepiness and drowsiness in America has been recognized for nearly 90 years but unfortunately very little has changed regarding its prevalence and impact on public health. The issue that has not been emphasized is the peripheral damage due to sleepy drivers. One might ask why it has taken so long for government and courts to act to protect the public. It seems unreasonable that sleep issues have been acknowledged for so many years, yet we are still without a universal mandate that drivers be accountable for the risks they take in driving sleepy.

Maggie's Law

A good example of the judicial system's failure or reluctance to acknowledge peripheral damage is the death of 20-year-old student Maggie McDonald in 1997. She was killed when a sleepy driver struck her automobile head on. The first trial of the driver ended in a deadlock. In the next trial, the driver received a suspended jail sentence and a $200 fine because at that time it was not against the law to fall asleep while driving. This remedy was totally unacceptable but did demonstrate how little education government and courts had concerning sleepiness and sleepy drivers. However, the family persisted in attaining justice and eventually the New Jersey Legislature enacted "Maggie's Law." The law was the first of its kind, making it illegal to drive while sleep-impaired in the state of New Jersey.[28,29] Should death occur, the law allows for a conviction of vehicular homicide if driving while sleep-deprived. Keep in mind that this outcome was not initiated due to pressure from sleep education specialists, or by concerned law enforcement, government, or public health officials, but through the dedication of Maggie McDonnell's family.

Despite the expected impact of Maggie's Law, there is still a lack of education about the significant dangers of driving while tired, drowsy, sleepy, or fatigued. However, a positive outcome of the New Jersey statute was that it placed employers at risk of corporate liability for drowsy driving accidents if employees were required to work excessively long hours, such as seen in commercial driving and medical training.[30–32] Fortunately, there are many US states that now have legislative bills pending or passed that address drowsy driving issues.[29]

THE NATIONAL COMMISSION ON SLEEP

An important positive step for sleep was accomplished in 1992 by William Dement, who was the Director of the National Commission on Sleep Disorders Research.[33] A report from this commission was submitted to the US Congress and cited that 40 million Americans were chronically affected by various sleep disorders and that an additional 20 to 30 million experience some sort of intermittent sleep-related problem. The report projected that by 2010, 79 million Americans would have difficulty falling asleep and nearly 40 million would experience debilitating EDS. By 2050, this was expected to increase to 100 million and 50 million, respectively. The report's projections for 2010 have been verified, at least in part, in a recent report by the Institute of Medicine[34] identifying that 50 to 70 million Americans have chronic sleep and wakefulness disorders. The burden of sleepiness that includes sleepy driving clearly continues to grow despite substantial and long-standing scientific evidence advocating the benefit of education and treatment. The problem will continue to grow unless the medical community, government officials, and society as a whole take responsibility and personal accountability for their role in the problem.

ALCOHOL VERSUS SLEEPY DRIVING: A COMPARATIVE MODEL

What may facilitate a better understanding of the potential risks of sleepy driving is the comparative model of driving under the influence of alcohol. Alcohol-related driving accidents have been a major focus of Mothers Against Drunk Driving (MADD), who intervened with national educational goals to reduce drunk-driving fatalities. Their strategy changed the national thinking over a 15-year period, which resulted in an enormous decrease in drunk-driving deaths.[35] We can learn from the experiences of this group because they have made significant strides in a short period of time. Sleepy drivers and drunk drivers exhibit a common finding, which is slowing of "reaction time" in a dose-response manner.[36] There are other commonalities they may share, such as decrements in neurocognitive functions and vigilance.[37,38] Peer-reviewed literature supports the fact that driving sleepy is the same as driving drunk.[19] This association brings attention to both dangerous activities (alcohol or sleepiness) separately or in combination. The specific outcomes of driving sleepy, driving drunk, or a combination of both is presented by knowledgeable researchers in this field. There are many excellent articles on this subject. Hence, only a limited number are presented here.

Dinges and Kribbs[36] reported that effects on simple reaction time effects are seen if alcohol and sleepiness are combined secondary to acceleration of habituation. These investigators showed that increasing alcohol levels or minimal sleep, or a combination of both could cause gross errors in judgment and attentiveness during driving. The importance of an adequate reaction time while driving could be life saving for the driver and others involved.

As a brief reminder, at a speed of 60 miles per hour an automobile will have traveled 88 ft in 1 second. It is not uncommon for sleepy drivers to have one-half to 1-second reaction time or more. A reaction time equal to or longer than 500 ms is defined as a "lapse." Lapses are extremely dangerous to any driver that is sleepy or under the influence of drugs or alcohol.

Dawson and Reid[39] reported that 17 hours of sleep deprivation (wakefulness) produces cognitive psychomotor performance (CPP) at a level that was equivalent to the performance impairments seen in blood alcohol concentrations (BAC) of 0.05%. At 24 hours of wakefulness CPP performance decreased to the same level as the performance of a BAC of 0.10%, which is well over the legal driving limit in many states.

Falleti and colleagues[40] examined cognitive impairment over 24 hours of sustained wakefulness and BAC of 0.05%, and found that fatigue from sleep caused more impairment than alcohol.

Roehrs and colleagues[41] examined dose-related sedative effects from sleep loss to those of ethanol. Sleep loss was 2.7 times more potent than ethanol in grams per kilogram in sedative effects. In addition, sleep loss reduced measures of the Multiple Sleep Latency Test (MSLT).

Roehrs and colleagues[42] also evaluated sleepiness with low-dose alcohol for simulated driving and divided performance attention, reporting on sleepiness and alcohol in simulated driving. The results showed that sleepiness and low-dose ethanol together impaired simulated driving. The investigators suggested it was possible that low breath ethanol concentrations (BEC) beyond the point of zero BEC could explain the incidence of driving accidents because sleepiness was also present.

Haraldsson and Akerstedt[43] reported from Sweden that drowsiness is a greater traffic hazard than alcohol and that drowsy driving is an underestimated risk factor in official statistics, as 15% to 30% of traffic accidents are related to drowsiness. Accidents while drowsy result in 3 times as many fatalities.

Powell and colleagues[44] reported on reaction time (RT) performance in OSA and alcohol-impaired controls. RTs were selected as a metric for evaluation because it is well known that RT is altered in unsafe alcohol consumption and sleepiness. This prospective study of a comparative model assessed alcohol-challenged normal subjects and subjects with OSA. Eighty healthy subjects performed 4 RT time trials using a validated psychomotor vigilance test (PVT) during which time breath alcohol concentrations (BrACs) were incrementally elevated to 0.08 g/dL or greater. The same PVT test was done on 113 subjects with OSA without alcohol. The OSA subjects had a mean respiratory disturbance index (RDI) of 29.2 events per hour of sleep. The findings of this study demonstrated that subjects with a mean age of 47 years with mild to moderate OSA had a worse RT test performance than healthy nonsleepy subjects with a mean age of 29 years and a BrAC that was illegally high for driving motor vehicles in the state of California.

Williamson and Feyer[45] compared the effects on performance of sleep deprivation and alcohol. Sleep deprivation of 17 to 19 hours showed that performance was equivalent or worse than a BAC of 0.05%. Response actions were 50% slower and accuracy was also lower than in those subjects with alcohol. This result suggested that sleep deprivation could compromise driving performance.

Powell and colleagues[19] continued to evaluate the comparative risks of drowsy driving and alcohol-impaired performances during a real-time study on track driving experience. This investigation was the first to include actual driving of a motor vehicle with the intention of assessing alcohol versus sleepiness while driving. This prospective cohort study included 16 healthy matched adult subjects with 50% being women. Two groups were identified: sleep-deprived and alcohol-challenged. The sleep-deprived group was further subdivided into an acute deprivation group and a chronic deprivation group. The acute group was sleep deprived for 24 hours (one night without sleep). The other subdivided group comprised chronic subjects, who slept 2 hours less than their usual sleep periods for 7 days. All subjects underwent baseline RT testing with a PVT device.

Each subject then drove on a closed course set up to test performance at the General Motors test track in Mesa, Arizona. Baseline data from that drive were collected for comparison with the final performance results for each subject (sleep-deprived and alcohol groups). Seven days later at the same time period as the baseline testing, the entire sequence was repeated for sleep deprivation or alcohol intake. The outcomes showed that there were no significant between-group differences in sleep-depravation or alcohol-intake groups before and after intervention for all 11 RT (PVT) tests. The magnitude of change was almost identical in both groups, even in light of the mean BAC of 0.089 g/dL in the alcohol group. On-track driving performance had similar results with a $P = .724$ when change scores for between groups were evaluated (baseline and at final driving). The overall outcome of the study could not be generalized because the subject numbers were small. However, the model suggests that there is a potential risk of driving sleepy that is at least as dangerous as driving illegally under the influence of alcohol.

The question is whether the general public is aware of these and the many other scientific investigations on driving sleepy, and whether without educational intervention they can be expected to make the correlation that driving sleepy is the same as driving drunk?

SLEEPY DRIVING ACCIDENT RISKS

The National Highway Traffic Safety Administration (NHTSA) and the National Center on Sleep Disorders Research (NCSDR) sponsored an expert panel on driver fatigue and sleepiness chaired by Strohl and colleagues.[24] This panel was a comprehensive effort to review the drowsy driving that has led to thousands of automobile accidents yearly. There were 7 sections from the introduction to the expert panel's recommendations. At completion, the panel suggested that there should be a focus on education concerning "drowsy driving," which included: education of young males, effective countermeasures, raising public awareness, educating shift workers, and education from other sectors. This study also covered crash characteristics and risks for drowsy driving crashes. The crash characteristics are summarized as follows: problems occur during late night and early morning, crashes are usually serious, single vehicle crash, occurs on high-speed roadway, no attempt to avoid crash, and the driver is alone. Population groups at the highest risk have been created based on crash reports. Three population groups exist: young males age 16 to 29, shift workers, and untreated sleep disorders. The risks of drowsy driving crashes are limited to inferential findings because there is presently no objective methodology for a clear-cut assessment of an individual's level of

sleepiness. However, the important educational metrics are: sleep loss, driving patterns especially from midnight to 6 AM, driving excessive miles yearly or hours a day, and driving longer without a break. Risk factors also include the use of sedative medications, unrecognized or untreated OSA, and alcohol usage. Many of these factors have cumulative effects.

Powell and colleagues[46] reported on sleepy driver near misses that may predict accident risks in a prospective cross-sectional study using an Internet survey with Dateline NBC News. The results from 35,217 subjects (88% of the sample of 39,825) are as follows: the risk of 1 accident increased from 23.2% if there were no near misses to a high of 44.5% in those with 4 or more near-miss sleepy accidents over a 3-year period. The Epworth Sleepiness Scale (ESS) had an independent association with a near miss or an accident. An increase of 1 unit of ESS score (of a maximum of 24) was associated with having a 4.4% increase of being involved in at least 1 accident ($P<.0001$). There was a dose response between sleepy near misses and an actual accident. Hence, sleepy near-miss accidents may be a precursor of an actual driving accident.

Accidents and Injuries

Shortly after the aforementioned NCSDR/NHTSA report by Strohl and colleagues,[24] Powell and colleagues[9] published findings on sleepy driving accidents and injury. This investigation evaluated the associated risk of driving sleepy with predictors of driving accidents and injury secondary to sleepiness. The study was a cross-sectional Internet-linked survey during a Dateline NBC news program on sleepy driving. An online national driving test used a 15-question quiz and from that quiz, subjects could voluntarily move on to a more detailed questionnaire of 64 questions. These questions were designed to elicit data on driving habits, sleepiness, accidents, and injuries during the last 3 years. Responses from 10,870 drivers were evaluated. Demographic characteristics were recorded. The ESS baseline score was 7.4 ± 4.2 for drivers without accidents and ranged to 12.7 ± 7.2 for drivers with 4 or more accidents $P<.0001$. Twenty-three percent of all respondents had 1 or more accident in a 3-year period. Among respondents who reported 4 or more accidents, a marked association was seen for the most recent accident to include injury ($P<.0001$). Sleep disorders were reported in 22.5% of all respondents, and in drivers that had more than 3 accidents the prevalence was higher, at 35% ($P = .002$). Six independent predictors of accidents were identified based on a stepwise ordered multiple logistic regression analysis, which kept the variable if the adjusted *P* value was less than 0.01. These 6 predictors were age, not married, ESS, annual miles driven, percentage driving at night, and consulted a medical professional because tired.

Connor and colleagues[47] from the University of Auckland, New Zealand designed a case study to evaluate whether sleepy driving causes crash injuries. This population-based control study included 571 drivers who were involved in crashes. At least one subject per driver was injured or killed in the crash. Acute sleepy driving increased the risk of crashing where a subject in the car was either injured or killed. There was no increase in risk associated with measures of chronic sleepiness.

SUMMARY

Acute and chronic sleepiness are pervasive in modern society, and are generally the result of volitional insufficient sleep or are secondary to an underlying sleep disorder. However, regardless of the cause of sleepiness, the outcome can cause human-error–related accidents and injuries due to decrements in neurobehavioral functions. These decrements may negatively affect RTs and vigilance to such a degree as to cause a motor vehicle accident and possible injury or death. The prevalence of sleepiness in our society has been reported to be as high as 33% and therefore there is an immense pool of sleepy driving subjects, many of whom ignore or are oblivious to the signs of sleepiness and persist to drive. We know from the large number of peer-review investigations that driving sleepy is the same as driving drunk. Unfortunately, we presently have no reasonable objective method to evaluate an unfit driver due to sleepiness alone. This may be, in large part, why efforts to teach the public about the dangers of sleepy driving have been relatively unsuccessful.

The risks of sleepy driving have very few legal sanctions and presently no objective testing methods. The scientific effort over numerous decades to better understand sleepiness and driving has also evaluated sleepiness risks in fields that require constant vigilance, for example, airlines, nuclear power, railroads, and medicine. We are still waiting for a method to assist in monitoring the levels of sleepiness and vigilance of motor vehicle drivers. This method should objectively assess sleepiness in much the same way as a breath or blood alcohol test evaluates alcohol levels.

Education, however, remains a critical element if change is to occur. Information about sleepiness and driving is readily available in the scientific literature, but it is not reaching the public in a way that they can relate to on a personal basis. Everyone who tests for a driver's license, in every state of the Union and every country of the world, should be able to answer basic questions about the signs of sleepiness and about the risks of driving sleepy. A point to consider is that if the medical literature contained data about a previously ignored disease that was now known to kill thousands of people each year, the news outlets would spread the word overnight. The dangers of sleepy driving need to receive similar, sustained attention.

REFERENCES

1. Ohayon MM, Caulet M, Philip P, et al. How sleep and mental disorders are related to complaints of daytime sleepiness. Arch Intern Med 1997;157: 2645–52.
2. Hublin C, Kaprio J, Partinen M, et al. Insufficient sleep—a population-based study in adults. Sleep 2001;24:392–400.
3. Bonnet M, Arand D. We are chronically sleep deprived. Sleep 1995;18:908–11.
4. Young T, Palta M, Dempsey J, et al. The occurrence of sleep disordered breathing among middle-aged adults. N Engl J Med 1993;328:1230–5.
5. Engleman H, Douglas N. Sleep-4: sleepiness, cognitive function, and quality of life in obstructive sleep apnoea/hypopnea syndrome. Thorax 2004; 59:618–22.
6. Durmer JS, Dinges DF. Neurocognitive consequences of sleep deprivation. Semin Neurol 2005; 25(1):117–29.
7. Young T, Blustein J, Finn L, et al. Sleep-disordered breathing and motor vehicle accidents in a population-based sample of employed adults. Sleep 1997;20(8):608–13.
8. Horne J, Reyner L. Vehicle accidents related to sleep: a review. Occup Environ Med 1999;56: 289–94.
9. Powell N, Schechtman K, Riley R, et al. Sleepy driving: accidents and injury. Otolaryngol Head Neck Surg 2002;126:217–27.
10. George C, Smiley A. Sleep apnea and automobile crashes. Sleep 1999;22(6):790–5.
11. Lyznicki J, Doege T, Davis R, et al. Sleepiness, driving, and motor vehicle crashes. JAMA 1998; 279:1908–13.
12. Maycock G. Sleepiness and driving: the experience of heavy goods vehicle drivers in the UK. J Sleep Res 1997;6:238–44.
13. Masa J, Rubio M, Findley L. Habitually sleepy drivers have a high frequency of automobile

crashes associated with respiratory disorders during sleep. Am J Respir Crit Care Med 2000; 162:1407–12.

14. National Transportation Safety Board [Internet]. Highway special investigation report medical oversight of noncommercial drivers. NTSB Number SIR-04/01. NTIS Number PB2004-917002. PDF Document. April 2001. Available at: http://www.ntsb.gov/publictn/2004/SIR0401.htm. Accessed November 16, 2004.

15. Drobnich D. A National Sleep Foundation's conference summary: the National Summit to prevent drowsy driving and a new call to action. Ind Health 2005;43:197–200.

16. Ohayon M. Prevalence and correlates of nonrestorative sleep complaints. Arch Intern Med 2005;165: 35–41.

17. Reyner L, Horne J. Falling asleep whilst driving: are drivers aware of prior sleepiness? Int J Legal Med 1998;111:120–3.

18. Dinges D, Mallis M. Managing fatigue by drowsiness detection. In: Hartley L, editor. Managing fatigue in transportation: Proceedings of the 3rd Fatigue in Transportation Conference, Fremantle, Western Australia, 1998. Western Australia: Institute for Research in Safety and Transport Murdoch University; 1998. p. 209–18.

19. Powell N, Schechtman K, Riley R, et al. The road to danger: the comparative risks of driving while sleepy. Laryngoscope 2001;111:887–93.

20. Akerstedt T, Kecklund G, Hörte L. Night driving, season, and the risk of highway accidents. Sleep 2001;24:401–6.

21. Pack AI, Pack AM, Rodgman E, et al. Characteristics of crashes attributed to the driver having fallen asleep. Accid Anal Prev 1995;27:769–75.

22. Stutts J, Wilkins J, Vaughn B. Why do people have drowsy driving crashes? Input from drivers who just did. Washington, DC: University of North Carolina School of Medicine for AAA Foundation for Traffic Safety; 1999.

23. Strohl K, Bonnie R, Findley L, et al. Sleep apnea, sleepiness, and driving risk. Am J Respir Crit Care Med 1994;150:1463–73.

24. Strohl K, Blatt J, Council F, et al. Drowsy driving and automobile crashes. Washington, DC: National Highway Traffic Safety Administration; 2001. Available at: http://www.nhtsa.dot.gov/PEOPLE/INJURY/drowsy_driving1/drowsy.html.

25. McComas HC. Controlling the airplane at twenty thousand feet, vol. 12. New York: Scientific Monthly; 1921. p. 36–46.

26. Mayer M. Report on human factor in the prevention of traffic accidents (French). International management congress, Washington (personal-general papers); 1938. p. 97–101.

27. Ellen RL, Marshal SC, Palayew M, et al. Systematic review of motor vehicle crash risk in persons with sleep apnea. J Clin Sleep Med 2006;2(2): 193–200.

28. New Jersey Legislature. Available at: http://www.njleg.state.nj.us/2002/Bills/A1500/1347_R2.HTM. Accessed February 10, 2003.

29. National Sleep Foundation. NSF statement regarding Maggie's law—nation's first law aimed at drowsy driving, May 2007.

30. Philip P, Taillarad J, Leger D, et al. Work and rest sleep schedules of 227 European truck drivers. Sleep Med 2002;3:507–11.

31. Barger L, Cade B, Ayas N, et al. Extended work shifts and the risk of motor vehicle crashes among interns. N Engl J Med 2005;352:125–34.

32. Pack AI, Maislin G, Staley B, et al. Impaired performance in commercial drivers role of sleep apnea and short sleep duration. Am J Respir Crit Care Med 2006;174:446–54.

33. National Commission on Sleep Disorders Research. Report of the National Commission on Sleep Disorders Research. Washington, DC: Superintendent of Documents, US Government Printing Office; 1992. Department of Health and Human Services Publication 92.

34. Institute of Medicine. Sleep disorders and sleep deprivation: an unmet public health problem. Washington, DC: National Academies Press; 2006.

35. National Highway Traffic Administration. Traffic safety facts 2007 data: alcohol impaired driving. DOT HS 810 985. PDF.2008. Washington, DC: National Highway Traffic Administration.

36. Dinges DF, Kribbs NB. Comparison of the effects of alcohol and sleepiness on simple reaction time performance: enhanced habituation as a common process. Alcohol Drugs Driving 1990; 5(4):329–39.

37. Kribbs NB, Dinges DF. Vigilance decrements and sleepiness. In: Hash JR, Ogilvie RD, editors. Sleep onset mechanisms. Washington, DC: American Psychological Association; 1994. p. 113–25.

38. Nicholson ME, Wang M, Collins O, et al. Variability in behavioral impairment involved in the rising and falling BAC curve. J Stud Alcohol 1992;53(4):349–56.

39. Dawson D, Reid K. Fatigue, alcohol and performance impairment. Nature 1997;388:235.

40. Falleti MG, Maruff P, Collie A, et al. Qualitative similarities in cognitive impairment associated with 24 h of sustained wakefulness and a blood alcohol concentration of 0.05%. J Sleep Res 2003;12:265–74.

41. Roehrs T, Burduvali E, Monahoom MA, et al. Ethanol and sleep loss: a "dose" comparison of impairing effects. Sleep 2003;26(8):981–5.

42. Roehrs T, Beare D, Zorick F, et al. Sleepiness and ethanol effects on simulated driving. Alcohol Clin Exp Res 1994;18(1):154–8.

43. Haraldsson PO, Akerstedt T. [Drowsiness-greater traffic hazard than alcohol. Causes, risks and treatment]. Lakartidningen 2001;98(25):3018–23 [in Swedish].

44. Powell NB, Riley RW, Schechtman KB, et al. A comparative model: reaction time performance in sleep-disordered breathing versus alcohol-impaired controls. Laryngoscope 1999;109:1648–54.

45. Williamson AM, Feyer AM. Moderate sleep deprivation produces impairments in cognitive and motor performance equivalent to legally prescribed levels of alcohol intoxication. Occup Environ Med 2000; 57:649–55.

46. Powell NB, Schechtman KB, Riley RW, et al. Sleepy driver near-misses may predict accident risks. Sleep 2007;30(3):331–42.

47. Connor J, Norton R, Ameratunga S, et al. Driver sleepiness and risk of serious injury to car occupants: population based case control study. BMJ 2002;324:1125.

Index

Note: Page numbers of article titles are in **boldface** type.

A

Accidents, risks due to sleepy driving, 121–122
Acetylcholine, role in neurology of sleep, 4–5
Adolescents, learning, memory, and sleep in, **45–57**
    correlational relationships between, 47–50
      disordered childhood sleep, 50
    development of sleep, 45–47
    direct comparisons of memory consolidation
      during wake and sleep, 51–53
    effects of sleep restriction on, 50–51
    neurocognitive effects of sleep disruption in,
      109–116
      common thread between, 114
      cultural, 109–110
      delayed sleep phase syndrome, 111
      narcolepsy, 113
      poor sleep hygiene/insufficient sleep, 110–111
      restless legs syndrome/periodic limb
        movement, 113
      sleep-disordered breathing, 111–113
        and ADHD, 112
        cognitive dysfunction, 112–113
        conduct disorder and aggressive behavior,
          112
Affect, sleep and emotional memory processing,
    31–43
Aggression, sleep-disordered breathing in children
    and, 112
Alcohol, driving under the influence compared with
    sleepy driving, 119–121
Animal models, sleep states and memory processing
    in rodents, **59–70**
Attention deficit hyperactivity disorder (ADHD), sleep-
    disordered breathing in children and, 112

B

Behavior, effects of sleep disruption in children and
    adolescents, **109–116**
    common thread between, 114
    cultural, 109–110
    delayed sleep phase syndrome, 111
    narcolepsy, 113
    poor sleep hygiene/insufficient sleep, 110–111
    restless legs syndrome/periodic limb
      movement, 113
    sleep-disordered breathing, 111–113
      and ADHD, 112

      cognitive dysfunction, 112–113
      conduct disorder and aggressive behavior,
        112
Brain stimulation, during sleep, **85–95**
    after TMS-induced plasticity, 92
    during SWS, 86–89
    historical perspective and stimulation
      protocols, 85–86
    memory and homeostatic regulation, 90–92
    TMS stimulation to probe brain excitability
      during, 89–90

C

cAMP, molecular basis for interactions between
    sleep and memory, **71–84**
cAMP response element binding protein, molecular
    basis for interactions between sleep and memory,
    71–84
Children, learning, memory, and sleep in, **45–57**
    correlational relationships between, 47–50
      children and adolescents, 49–50
      disordered childhood sleep, 50
      infants, 47–49
    development of sleep, 45–47
      adolescence, 47
      early and middle childhood, 46–47
      gestational sleep, 45
      neonatal and infant sleep, 46
    direct comparisons of memory consolidation
      during wake and sleep, 51–53
    effects of sleep restriction on, 50–51
    neurocognitive effects of sleep disruption in,
      109–116
      common thread between, 114
      cultural, 109–110
      delayed sleep phase syndrome, 111
      narcolepsy, 113
      poor sleep hygiene/insufficient sleep, 110–111
      restless legs syndrome/periodic limb
        movement, 113
      sleep-disordered breathing, 111–113
        and ADHD, 112
        cognitive dysfunction, 112–113
        conduct disorder and aggressive behavior,
          112
      treatment of sleep problems, 113
Circadian rhythm, control of sleep-dependent
    memory processing, 77–78

Circadian rhythm (*continued*)
  in neurology of sleep, 8−9
    clock genes, 9
    homeostatic and circadian sleep-wake
      interactions, 9−10
    suprachiasmatic nucleus, 8−9
Cognition, experiencing consolidation of memory,
  sleep and dreaming, **97−108**
Cognitive dysfunction, sleep-disordered breathing
  in children and, 112−113
Cognitive outcomes, learning, memory, and sleep
  in children, **45−57**
Conduct disorder, sleep-disordered breathing
  in children and, 112
Consolidation, of memory, sleep and dreaming,
  97−108
Cultural factors, in determining normal sleep
  in children, 109−110

D

Delayed sleep phase syndrome, in children and
  adolescents, 111
Depression, sleep and emotional memory
  processing, 36−38
Disrupted sleep. *See* Sleep disruption.
Dopamine, role in neurology of sleep, 6
Dreaming, experiencing consolidation of sleep and
  memory and, **97−108**
    empirical study of spontaneous subjective
      experience, 104−105
    incorporation of recent experience into,
      100−104
      determinants of memory sources of,
        101−102
      effects of intensive learning experiences
        on sleep onset mentation, 102
      effects of presleep experience on sleep
        mentation, 100−101
      interleaved fragments of experience,
        102−104
    memories in the sleeping brain, 97−100
      linking sleep-dependent memory
        processing with dream experience,
        99−100
      reactivation and consolidation, 97−99
      reactivation of memory in dream content,
        105−106
Driving, sleepiness and, **117−124**
  accident risks, 121−122
  brief review, 117
  compared with driving under the influence
    of alcohol, 119−121
  history of, Maggie's law, 119
    problem of, 119
    what has now been accomplished,
      118−119

what was previously accomplished, 118
National Commission on Sleep, 119
Drowsiness, and driving, **117−124**

E

Electroencephalogram (ECG), brain stimulation
  during sleep, **85−95**
Emotional memory processing, sleep and, **31−43**
  affective memory consolidation, 34−35
  affective memory encoding, 32−34
  emotional regulation, 35−36
  heuristic model of sleep-dependent emotional
    processing, 38
  sleep loss, mood stability, and emotional brain
    (ro)activity, 36−38
  sleep to forget and sleep to remember
    hypothesis, 38−41
Entrainment, agents of, in neurology of sleep, 11−12
  light, 11
  melatonin, 11−12

F

Forced desynchrony, in neurology of sleep, 10−11

G

Genetic models, to study sleep−memory
  interactions, 79
Gestational sleep, development of, 45

H

Hippocampus, sleep's role in memory processing
  and storing in humans, **15−30**
Histamine, role in neurology of sleep, 6
Homeostatic regulation, brain stimulation during
  sleep and memory, 90−91
  in control of sleep-dependent memory
    processing, 77−78
  in neurology of sleep, 9−10
Hygiene, sleep. See Sleep hygiene.
Hypocretin, role in neurology of sleep, 6−8

I

Infants, correlational relationships between sleep and
  learning in, 47−49
  development of sleep in, 46
Insufficient sleep, in children and adolescents,
  110−111

L

Learning, and memory and sleep in children, **45−57**
  correlational relationships between, 47−50

children and adolescents, 49—50
disordered childhood sleep, 50
infants, 47—49
development of sleep, 45—47
adolescence, 47
early and middle childhood, 46—47
gestational sleep, 45
neonatal and infant sleep, 46
direct comparisons of memory consolidation
during wake and sleep, 51—53
effects of sleep restriction on, 50—51
molecular basis for interactions between sleep
and memory, **71—84**
Light, as agent of entrainment, 11

M

Maggie's Law, on driving while sleep impaired, 119
Melatonin, as agent of entrainment, 11—12
Memory, and learning and sleep in children, **45—57**
correlational relationships between, 47—50
children and adolescents, 49—50
disordered childhood sleep, 50
infants, 47—49
development of sleep, 45—47
adolescence, 47
early and middle childhood, 46—47
gestational sleep, 45
neonatal and infant sleep, 46
direct comparisons of memory consolidation
during wake and sleep, 51—53
effects of sleep restriction on, 50—51
brain stimulation during sleep and homeostatic
regulation, 90—92
emotional memory processing and sleep, **31—43**
affective memory consolidation, 34—35
affective memory encoding, 32—34
emotional regulation, 35—36
heuristic model of sleep-dependent emotional
processing, 38
sleep loss, mood stability, and emotional brain
(re)activity, 36—38
sleep to forget and sleep to remember
hypothesis, 38—41
experiencing consolidation of sleep and dreaming
and, **97—108**
empirical study of spontaneous subjective
experience, 104—105
incorporation of recent experience into
dreaming, 100—104
determinants of memory sources of
dreaming, 101—102
effects of intensive learning experiences
on sleep onset mentation, 102
effects of presleep experience on sleep
mentation, 100—101

interleaved fragments of experience,
102—104
memories in the sleeping brain, 97—100
linking sleep-dependent memory
processing with dream experience,
99—100
reactivation and consolidation, 97—99
reactivation of memory in dream content,
105—106
molecular basis for interaction between sleep and,
71—84
homeostatic and circadian control of sleep-
dependent memory processing, 77—78
molecular replay and sleep-dependent
memory processing, 78—79
sleep states and memory, 76—77
non-REM, 76—77
REM, 77
stages of memory processing, 71—76
acquisition/encoding, 72
retrieval and reconsolidation, 75
synaptic consolidation, 72—75
systems consolidation, 75
use of genetic models to study, 79
sleep states and memory processing in rodents,
59—70
future directions, 67
memory enhancement, 61—62
neurochemical and genetic factors, 65—67
acetylcholine, 65—66
intracellular mechanisms, 66—67
REM sleep and memory, 60—61
REM sleep and replay, 64—65
REM sleep generator, 61
status of sleep-memory theories, 67
SWS and memory, 62
SWS and replay, 62—64
sleep's role in, in humans, **15—30**
beyond sleep stages, 24
defining sleep and, 15—16
future directions, 27
neurophysiological and neurochemical
evidence for sleep's role in, 24—25
neurotransmitters and neurohormones,
25—27
sleep's benefits to emotional memory
consolidation, 22
sleep's benefits to explicit memories, 21—22
sleep's benefits to implicit and procedural
memories, 16—21
transformation of, 23—24
Mentation, experiencing consolidation of memory,
sleep and dreaming, **97—108**
Molecular studies, of interaction between sleep and
memory, **71—84**
homeostatic and circadian control of sleep-
dependent memory processing, 77—78

Molecular studies (*continued*)
    molecular replay and sleep-dependent
      memory processing, 78–79
    sleep states and memory, 76–77
      non-REM, 76–77
      REM, 77
    stages of memory processing, 71–76
      acquisition/encoding, 72
      retrieval and reconsolidation, 75
      synaptic consolidation, 72–75
      systems consolidation, 75
    use of genetic models to study, 79
Monoaminergic systems, role in neurology of sleep,
    5–6
Mood stability, sleep loss and emotional brain (re)
    activity, 36–38

N

Narcolepsy, neurocognitive effects in children and
    adolescents, 113
National Commission on Sleep, and sleepy driving,
    119
Neonates, development of sleep in, 46
Neurocognitive effects, of sleep disruption in children
    and adolescents, **109–116**
    common thread between, 114
    cultural, 109–110
    delayed sleep phase syndrome, 111
    narcolepsy, 113
    poor sleep hygiene/insufficient sleep, 110–111
    restless legs syndrome/periodic limb
      movement, 113
    sleep-disordered breathing, 111–113
      and ADHD, 112
      cognitive dysfunction, 112–113
      conduct disorder and aggressive behavior,
        112
Neurohormones, role in memory consolidation,
    25–27
Neurology, of sleep, **1–14**
    agents of entrainment, 11–12
      light, 11
      melatonin, 11–12
    ascending reticular system, 4–8
      acetylcholine, 4–5
      dopamine, 6
      hypocretin (orexin), 6–8
      monoaminergic systems, 5–6
      norepinephrine and histamine, 6
      serotonin, 6
    circadian rhythm, 8–9
      clock genes, 9
      suprachiasmatic nucleus, 8–9
    forced desynchrony, 10–11
    historical context, 1–2

homeostatic and circadian sleep-wake
      interactions, 9–10
    sleep and wake states, 2–4
Neurotransmitters, role in memory consolidation,
    25–27
Non-rapid eye movement (NREM) sleep, brain
    stimulation during, 86–91
    molecular basis for sleep–memory interactions,
      76–77
Norepinephrine, role in neurology of sleep, 6

O

Orexin, role in neurology of sleep, 6–8
Oscillation, in molecular basis for sleep-memory
    interactions, **71–84**
    slow, brain stimulation during non-REM sleep,
      86–93

P

Periodic limb movements, neurocognitive effects
    in children and adolescents, 113
Post-traumatic stress disorder (PTSD), sleep and
    emotional memory processing, 36–38
Protein kinase A, molecular basis for interactions
    between sleep and memory, **71–84**

R

Rapid eye movement (REM) sleep, and memory
    processing in rodents, **59–70**
    emotional memory processing and, **31–43**
    molecular basis for sleep–memory interactions,
      77
    role in processing and storing memories, **15–30**
Restless legs syndrome, neurocognitive effects in
    children and adolescents, 113
Reticular activating system, in neurology of sleep,
    4–8
    acetylcholine, 4–5
    dopamine, 6
    hypocretin (orexin), 6–8
    monoaminergic systems, 5–6
    norepinephrine and histamine, 6
    serotonin, 6
Rodents, sleep states and memory processing in,
    59–70
    future directions, 67
    memory enhancement, 61–62
    neurochemical and genetic factors, 65–67
      acetylcholine, 65–66
      intracellular mechanisms, 66–67
    REM sleep and memory, 60–61
    REM sleep and replay, 64–65
    REM sleep generator, 61

status of sleep-memory theories, 67
SWS and memory, 62
SWS and replay, 62–64

S

School achievement, learning, memory, and sleep
  in children, **45–57**
Serotonin, role in neurology of sleep, 6
Sleep, and memory and learning, 1–124
  brain stimulation during, **85–95**
    after TMS-induced plasticity, 92
    during SWS, 86–89
    historical perspective and stimulation
      protocols, 85–86
    memory and homeostatic regulation,
      90–92
    TMS stimulation to probe brain excitability
      during, 89–90
  emotional memory processing and, **31–43**
    heuristic model of sleep-dependent
      emotional processing, 38
    sleep loss, mood stability, and emotional
      brain (re)activity, 36–38
    sleep to forget and sleep to remember
      hypothesis, 38–41
  experiencing consolidation of memory, sleep
    and dreaming, **97–108**
    empirical study of spontaneous subjective
      experience, 104–105
    incorporation of recent experience into
      dreaming, 100–104
    memories in the sleeping brain, 97–100
    reactivation of memory in dream content,
      105–106
  in children, **45–57**
    correlational relationships between, 47–50
    development of sleep, 45–47
    direct comparisons of memory
      consolidation during wake and sleep,
      51–53
    effects of sleep restriction on, 50–51
  in rodents, **59–70**
    future directions, 67
    memory enhancement, 61–62
    neurochemical and genetic factors, 65–67
    REM sleep and memory, 60–61
    REM sleep and replay, 64–65
    REM sleep generator, 61
    SWS and memory, 62
    SWS and replay, 62–64
  molecular basis for interaction between,
    71–84
    homeostatic and circadian control of sleep-
      dependent memory processing, 77–78
    molecular replay and sleep-dependent
      memory processing, 78–79

sleep states and memory, 76–77
stages of memory processing, 71–76
use of genetic models to study, 79
neurocognitive effects of sleep disruption
  in children and adolescents, **109–116**
    common thread between, 114
    cultural, 109–110
    delayed sleep phase syndrome, 111
    narcolepsy, 113
    poor sleep hygiene/insufficient sleep,
      110–111
    restless legs syndrome/periodic limb
      movement, 113
    sleep-disordered breathing, 111–113
    treatment of sleep problems, 113
neurology of, agents of entrainment, 11–12
  ascending reticular system, 4–8
  circadian rhythm, 8–9
  forced desynchrony, 10–11
  historical context, 1–2
  homeostatic and circadian sleep-wake
    interactions, 9–10
  sleep and wake states, 2–4
role in memory processing and storing in
  humans, **15–30**
  benefits to emotional memory
    consolidation, 22
  benefits to explicit memories, 21–22
  benefits to implicit and procedural
    memories, 16–21
  beyond sleep stages, 24
  defining sleep and memory, 15–16
  future directions, 27
  neurophysiological and neurochemical
    evidence for sleep's role in, 24–25
  neurotransmitters and neurohormones,
    25–27
  transformation of memories, 23–24
sleepy driving, **117–124**
Sleep apnea, sleepy driving due to, **117–124**
Sleep disruption, neurocognitive effects in children
  and adolescents, **109–116**
    common thread between, 114
    cultural, 109–110
    delayed sleep phase syndrome, 111
    narcolepsy, 113
    poor sleep hygiene/insufficient sleep,
      110–111
    restless legs syndrome/periodic limb
      movement, 113
    sleep-disordered breathing, 111–113
      and ADHD, 112
      cognitive dysfunction, 112–113
      conduct disorder and aggressive behavior,
        112
Sleep hygiene, poor, in children and adolescents,
  110–111

Sleep-disordered breathing, in children and
    adolescents, 111–113
        and ADHD, 112
        cognitive dysfunction and, 112–113
        conduct disorder and aggressive behavior, 112
Sleepiness, and driving, **117–124**
        accident risks, 121–122
        brief review, 117
        compared with driving under the influence
            of alcohol, 119–121
        history of, 117–119
        National Commission on Sleep, 119

Slow wave sleep (SWS), and memory processing
    in rodents, **59–70**
    role in processing and storing memories, **15–30**
    stimulating the brain during, 86–89
Stimulation. *See* Brain stimulation.

T

Transcranial direct current (DC) stimulation, during
    sleep, **85–95**
Transcranial magnetic stimulation (TMS), during
    sleep, **85–95**

Printed and bound by CPI Group (UK) Ltd, Croydon, CR0 4YY

03/10/2024

01040350-0016

Moving?

Make sure your subscription moves with you!

To notify us of your new address, find your **Clinics Account Number** (located on your mailing label above your name), and contact customer service at:

Email: journalscustomerservice-usa@elsevier.com

800-654-2452 (subscribers in the U.S. & Canada)
314-447-8871 (subscribers outside of the U.S. & Canada)

Fax number: 314-447-8029

Elsevier Health Sciences Division
Subscription Customer Service
3251 Riverport Lane
Maryland Heights, MO 63043

ELSEVIER